Essential Connections

The How & Why of Your Personal Energy

By

Felicity Rose Mackinnon

Published by
Adeline Ink

~

Adeline Ink.
Hampshire, England.

'Essential Connections'
The How & Why Of Your Personal Energy.

Catalogue record for this book is available from the British Library.

Watercolours and graphics by the Author.
Additional graphics by Joshua Torr.
Cover design by Kim Hills.

ISBN 978-178035-264-0

First published 2012 by ADELINE INK.
Printed by FASTPRINT PUBLISHING
Peterborough, England.

This is for my beloved Mama,
and dedicated to my much-loved family.

About the Author.

An early background in nursing and then learning energy healing through Reiki years later, led the author to seek much deeper knowledge and understanding of the body. Discovering the gulf between scientific books on anatomy and the metaphysical works on energy and the chakras, prompted a strong desire to combine the two in one book. This then became a passionate belief in the need for these two to be seen and understood as not separate fields at all, but one: they are inextricably combined in the whole person. This led to a profound and exciting writing odyssey for this book.
She lives in Hampshire and is busy continuing with her writing.

Acknowledgements.

First all my loving thanks to my wonderful children and my sisters, for their total belief in me and support for my book. Warm thanks also to my friend Sheila for her recognition and belief in the need for this book from the beginning. They have all encouraged and sustained me *so* much. Thanks go also to all my friends who have patiently listened to me on the subject over the years!

From the Author

The body you have is the one your 'Self', your personality, the 'You' lives within. It will give you all the experiences, joys and sorrows of your lifetime. People and events will come and go, but you and your body will be together still.

It is therefore valuable to you…so you must get to know it, treat it well, help it all you can and above all, appreciate, even love the substance of it, because 'you' are within.

I have written this book for you to get to know the workings of your body and the source of your emotions….for it is these two together that make up the quality of your life….for good or ill. Once you understand the reasons 'why' of these vital aspects, you will truly be able to have a care for yourself which will show in a happier, healthier and more empathetic you. First and foremost *you* will benefit, ….and others will, simply as a consequence of your understanding of yourself, and of other people's ways of being.

The emotions that we hurt ourselves with give us memories that keep coming back to haunt and taunt us. We need to dissolve those emotional ties that let this happen so that memories are what they should be, reminders for future reference. Here in this book I will show you how. It really is in your power to make life happier and healthier. Once you know how you create the energy within you from the emotions you carry, you can decide to transform it to enrich your life.

I offer this book to you with genuine heartfelt wishes that you can find more enjoyment, better health and peace of mind in this stressful life, just as I have from all I have learned in writing it.

Be yourself.
Your self is within.
Treasure it as the place where knowledge 'is',
'will come to',…
and will expand the true Self into a loving human being.

Felicity Rose Mackinnon.

Contents.

Section 1. The Body.

This first section is to offer a new perspective on your body.

It explores the functions and processes of those organs which are most involved with how our energy is created through the core of the body. The most relevant to our energy, as you will see, is the endocrine or hormonal system which controls the whole body in amazing ways. However, some other organs are closely involved with them so are highly relevant too. The energy produced is made up of our physical and mental activities and the emotional energy we generate.

The body and mind work together in a constant relationship. While our thoughts stimulate our emotional energy it is the body that responds and expresses them. Our energy is a most precious commodity. It is knowing how and why it works that will help us enormously with life's challenges, experiences and relationships.

It is within the anatomy and physiology of the specialised and amazing organs we are exploring that we can find the sources of our emotional energy. Our emotions are related to their functions. To this end, after each organ or area that has been explored, the sources of the thoughts and feelings that are likely to arise are set out. These chapter sections are about the associated Energy Centres (also known as chakras) from which our energy is circulated. These are where emotional energy collects. Thus through our anatomical functions we can discover the effects emotions have on the body's whole energy system and ultimately, the state of our health.

By knowing the physical 'how' and 'why' of the anatomy it is much easier to understand 'why' and 'how' our bodies work for us and how emotional energy affects its functions. Once we see the logical connections of our anatomy, its physiology and our emotions, we can better understand ourselves and others. With these insights we can really take a hand in our own health and improve the quality of life, and also our personal development for better relationships.

All the anatomy is easy to read and each chapter is set out to be referred to again and again. Your memory can be frequently refreshed and you can check up and explore any particular aspect at a later date. For ready access each anatomy chapter has its own glossary of anatomical terms and words used. There is also a full glossary at the end of the book.

To help you with this there are Personal Notes pages set aside for your use after each chapter. Anything that you recognise, relate to or reminds you of something etc can be jotted down as you go. Making use of these pages will be invaluable.

Any uncertainty about what we are feeling and why can be very stressful in itself. 'Not knowing' leads to needless anxiety. Any knowledge that reduces the kind of stress that undermines our peace of mind and our health is essential if we are to cope well with the pressures of modern life. Know your body and you can always help yourself.

Chapter 1. An Introduction to Essential Anatomy.

In this section we will explore the core of the body through the inner world of its anatomy and physiology. But first, a look at the overall functionality of the Endocrine System. This is where we are going to start because it influences the entire body and interacts with your emotions. Then we'll look at its individual organs. The endocrine or hormone system is comprised of a series of small, specialised ductless glands. These produce and secrete the vital hormones necessary *to regulate the whole body.* Each gland is in constant touch with the master gland, the *pituitary*, in an inter-linked and inter-related relationship with its own regulatory system of checks and balances.

It is this balancing regulatory function that makes it the most relevant in complementary healing approaches.

The function of this endocrine hormonal system is to keep in balance all the other systems so that together they enable the body to work efficiently as a harmonious whole. This state of balance is called *homeostasis*. As soon as there is an imbalance the appropriate hormones are produced and released or inhibited to correct it as quickly as possible because this maintains and sustains good health.

Homeostasis:……(Greek*: homoios* = 'the same' = *stasis* = 'standing').

This is the **constancy** of the body's internal condition for healthy function. If this is upset or unbalanced, the system has a specialised system of **negative feedback** mechanisms to return the body to normal. If the upset and disturbance goes beyond the fluctuations of everyday life, which the normal healthy body can easily deal with, then conditions of illness or disease have developed. The general health, the effects, and seriousness of the condition will be relative factors.

acute (short-term) illness:
the body can be restored to homeostasis fairly quickly.

chronic (long-term) illness:
when the endocrine system is unable to return the body to normal internal condition then this will indicate serious disease.

If homeostasis cannot be restored at all, the body will close down.

Under the headings of '*what*', '*where*' '*how*' and '*why*' we will look at the workings of the system through the structure and function of the glands in it. Their processes are all part of the energy system that keeps us in good health.

The pale orange boxes contain factual information and in the main the turquoise boxes give observations and insights. All these are to make it easy for checking back, refreshing your memory or for future needs as a ready reference. After each anatomy section in Chapters 1- 9, you will find a glossary of terms to help you as you go along in case you need it. There is also a full glossary at the end. There will be little helpful anecdotes and notes along the way as well.

There are 7 solely ductless endocrine glands. However the Pancreas is dealt with here with the endocrine system although not strictly an endocrine gland. But, because its main function is to provide the sugar-regulator hormone Insulin it can be classed with the rest since Insulin enters the blood via diffusion. The Pancreas also has a digestive function but a duct is used for these secretions.

Essential to the functioning of the endocrine hormonal system is the co-ordination and partnership of the nervous system, the ***neuro-endocrine*** system, which enables all the fine adjustments to be made to maintain homeostasis.

In order to understand this neural partnership, we will look at the upper brain and the areas that relay and co-ordinate instructions to keep everything humming along. Also running down the midline is the **A**utonomic **N**ervous **S**ystem which we'll explore too. This is the system that runs the internal organs. Lastly we'll look at the spinal nerves which supply the periphery of the body, and their destination, the sensory dermatomes.

Thus we will discover the regulation of the inside and outside of the body fully, from its central core.

Two major organs closely involved with the endocrine system are the liver and spleen. They play a large part in the vital energy system that deals with our health and well-being that we are exploring here. Their particular functions and processes are therefore important to complete the picture as we move down through the body.

We will now start with the Endocrine System itself.

******

The Endocrine System.

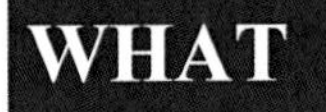

Endocrinology is the study of the **structure** and **function** of the endocrine glands and the hormones that they **produce**, **store** and **secrete.**

This is a co-ordinated interlocking relationship and affects practically all cell activity. It is therefore responsible for *tissue activity* throughout the body.

HOW

Hormones: (Greek.'*active within*')............'excite' or activate, tissue activity.

The glands where they originate are *ductless*; the hormones are released directly into the bloodstream by *diffusion* from Secretory cells.

- These have specialised 'gates' in the cell wall; hormones pass through into the interstitial fluid in extracellular (*extra* = outside. *cellular* = 'of a cell') spaces around the secretory cells themselves.
- Hormones then pass through single-cell walls of tiny blood capillaries into bloodstream.
- Blood flows very slowly in capillaries so gives necessary time for sufficient molecules to diffuse into the blood.

A considerable network of surrounding tiny blood capillaries therefore, supplies the glands. The hormones are then carried into the main bloodstream for dispersal.
Each one is attracted by special protein cell receptors waiting just inside the cells in the appropriate organ.

Each hormone fulfils its appropriate and specialised function **in that cell only**.
Hormone and receptor lock together and produce the necessary chemical reaction.

Some hormones are local to their point of origin, some are circulating hormones. Some of these float in the bloodstream in a dormant state waiting to be triggered when necessary. Most disperse to all cells in the body.

Surplus and used hormones are *re-cycled* through the liver. (*See* Liver p94)
& excreted via the kidneys.
In kidney/liver failure they can build up causing further tissue stress.

WHY

Balance throughout the body has to be maintained:
to ensure correct hormone levels.

- For appropriate hormonal secretion.
- For the correct timing of hormonal operation for proper function.
- In the number of hormones secreted.
- In the number of receptors within the cells awaiting hormone triggering.

This delicate balance is maintained by *modifying, delaying* or *with-holding* hormone activity as a counter to the activity required; a system of 'increase' and 'decrease' triggering off each other to ensure that all cell activity works as it should. The body's negative feedback mechanism constantly corrects this vital balance. *In this way all the systems of the body are able to function properly.*

Negative Feedback.
Once a specific hormone has been stimulated to correct an imbalance it needs to stop production once balance is achieved, so either the correctly balanced chemicals switch off the hormone production, or a specific 'inhibiting' hormone is released.

The endocrine system's **primary objective.**
By regulating the other systems it makes certain that they in turn ensure that the endocrine system can function correctly. This reciprocity indicates the inter-dependent relationship of the body as a whole unit.

WHAT

General Effects.

The Endocrine system:
Changes metabolic activities.
Regulates immune system & glandular secretions.
Regulates condition and volume of all extracellular fluid.
Regulates growth and development.
Guides & **induces** reproductive processes.

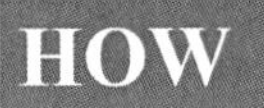

Through the <u>ENDOCRINE GLANDS</u> themselves.

A fascinating series of small highly active glands tucked into the protective cavities of the head and torso which we will look at in detail in the next section. (*See also* **Fig:1**.)

The Pineal. (or The Pineal Body)	**Brain cavity.**
The Pituitary. (two lobes: the anterior and posterior.)	**Brain cavity.**
The Thyroid. paired with; **The Parathyroid.**	**In the throat.**
The Thymus.	**Chest cavity.**
(The Pancreas.	*Abdominal cavity).*
The Adrenals.. (or The Suprarenals.)	**Abdominal cavity.**
The Ovaries and Testes.	**Pelvic cavity.**

WHERE

The **Pineal** and **Pituitary**, lie within the brain itself under the cerebrum.
The **Thyroid** lies in front of the trachea. (windpipe)
The **4 Parathyroids** are embedded in the thyroid towards the back of the trachea.
The **Thymus** lies under the sternum (breastbone) on top of the heart.
The **Adrenals** lie under the diaphragm and sit on top of the kidneys.) Known also as the Suprarenals: supra=above; renal=kidney)
The **Pancreas** lies between the kidneys; under the liver & stomach.
The **Ovaries** lie in the pelvic cavity, approximately level with the ileac crest. (Upper curve of hipbone)
The **Testes** lie outside the body in the scrotum for temperature control, but are *involuntarily* drawn up close to the body by the release of adrenalin from the Adrenals in cold temperatures to maintain the correct temperature for sperm production.

These small and highly influential endocrine glands are deeply embedded for the most part as they follow the core or centre line of the body. (*See* **Fig:1.**) The thyroid and parathyroids are possibly vulnerable but the strong complex neck muscles form a good protection.

Here we can see that the hormonal Endocrine glands follow the core of the body.

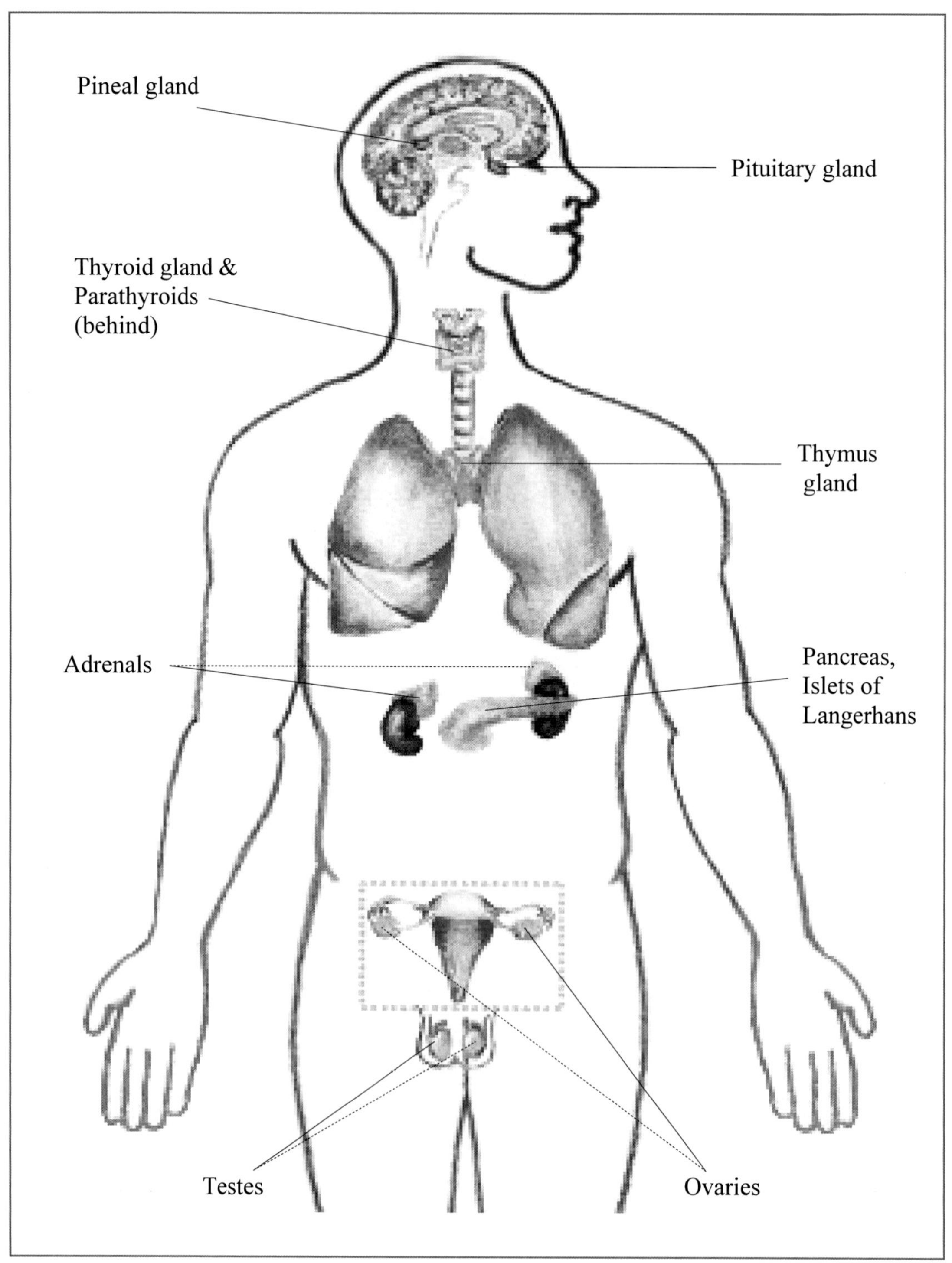

Fig:1. The Endocrine Glands.

The control of hormone **production, secretion** and also their **inhibition** is from *three* sources.

HOW

1) Impulses from the nervous system.
2) Chemical changes in the blood, eg: saline and glucose.
3) Other hormones.

All hormonal *activity* is stimulated in *two* ways.

1) Hormonal stimulation:.....works through the blood stream**.**
2) Neuronal stimulation:......works from muscular action and thought processes**.**

***Hormonal* Activity and Response.**
The effect is *long lasting.*
Can range between seconds and several hours for the required effect for:-
- sexual development.
- maintenance of reproductivity.
- metabolism of nutrients.
- balance of blood chemicals.

***Neurone* activity and response.**
is *short-lived.* Consistently rapid for:-
- muscular action.
- thought processes.

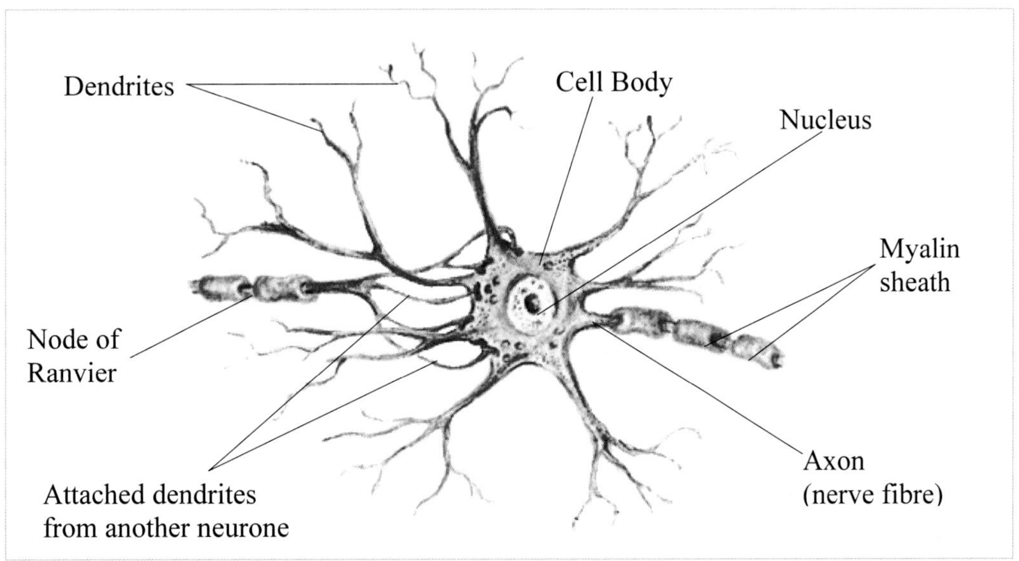

Fig:2. Neurone: nerve cell plus axon.

Glossary.

Anterior:…At or to the front.
Axon:…nerve fibre; can be any length up to 3 feet.
Posterior:...At or to the back.
Capillaries:…tiny vessels carrying fluids (blood or lymph) from tissues to arteries and veins.
Diffusion:…to pass directly through the cell walls. (always from an area of *greatest* concentration to one with less)
Dispersal:…spread out to other areas.
Ductless:…has no collecting tube (duct) to carry substances to other areas.
Endocrine:…Gk; *endo* = inside; *krinein* = secrete.
Glucose:…simplified sugar. Small enough molecules for absorption.
Hormone:…alters the physiological activity of target cells.
Hormonal:…hormone activity.
Impulses:…nerve messages that travel along nerve fibres to initiate action.
Inhibits/inhibition:…put an end or stop to.
Initiates:…starts off/sets in motion.
Metabolic:…chemical changes that manage energy throughout body.
Myalin:…fatty insulation formed from special neuroglia cells to conduct impulses.
Neural:…to do with nerves & their activity.
Neurone:…nerve cell (neuron) and nerve fibre (axon) together.
Nodes of Ranvier:…gaps in myalin sheath for nerve impulse to jump to increase speed
Trachea:…(tra..*kee*..a)…windpipe from throat to lungs.
Receptors:…cells that receive specific chemicals. Numbers increased & reduced as needed.
Saline:…salt in solution. (water)
Secretion:…useful fluid product made and released from a gland or cell.
Secretory:…has the ability to secrete specialised substances.
Schwann cells:…name for coils of myalin between nodes of Ranvier.
Stimulus:…a trigger to start activity.

NB. The over-secretion and under-secretion of all hormones produces adverse conditions and diseases in themselves. However the study of these is a separate issue

******

Chapter 2. The Pineal Gland. (epiphysis cerebri)

This is the first endocrine gland to look at as it is the uppermost in the body.
It is considered to be the body's 'biological' clock. Not everything is fully known about it, but it is a very important gland. Its functions are closely connected to emotion.

WHERE

This tiny cone-shaped gland (named for its resemblance to a pine cone) is situated behind the thalamus and hypothalamus (which make up the diencephalon: *see* p30). It is tucked neatly up under the third ventricle of the brain, a slit-like space, centred under the cerebrum and filled with cerebro-spinal fluid. The gland has a protective capsule around it made from the *pia mater*. one of the linings, or meninges, of the brain.

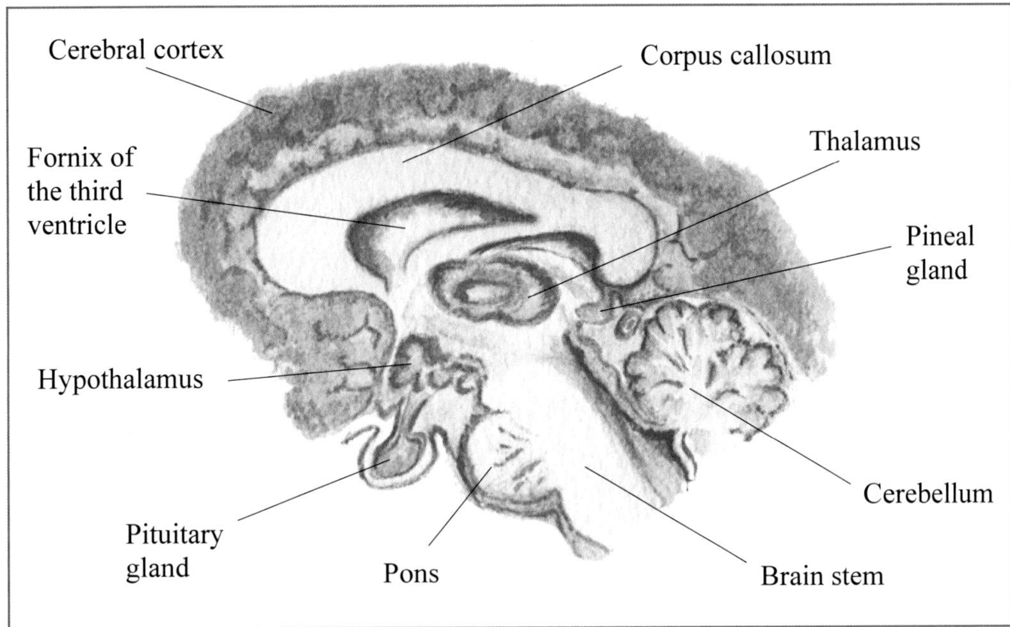

Fig:3. Sagittal view of centre of brain.

WHAT

Melatonin is the known hormone it produces & secretes.

The gland contains:-

- **Secretory** cells called **pinealocytes** for hormone production and release.
- Masses of **neuroglia**; for neural response primarily from optic nerve.
- **Seratonin**; inhibitory neurotransmitter; works with melatonin for sleep. It also balances emotions and moods and counters the fear response.*

HOW

Melatonin is secreted directly into the blood stream through the tiny blood capillaries supplying the gland.

Melatonin acts as a cerebral anæsthetic and is started and stopped *neurologically* by levels of *darkness* and *light* respectively, through the **optic nerve** which supplies the eye.

The response is in the neuroglia masses which are areas of supporting nervous tissue around the secretory cells. Thus the stimulus is from the *nervous system.* Neuro-secretory tissue is derived from cells detached from the sympathetic ganglia, an area of the brain. These cells develop in and into different organs. This connection means that the secretions are readily stimulated by nervous impulses because they originate from the same place. Seratonin, an inhibitory *neuro*tranmitter synthesised from proteins is found here in high concentration in the Pineal.

Seratonin acts to calm and balance the mind.
Counterbalances the fear response* from the adrenals, restoring the normal mood after the stimulus has passed. (*See* p137)

Seratonin levels are *low* in Clinical Depression.
It is used in Anti-depressants.

Darkness *increases* melatonin and secretion levels.
Light i*nterrupts* production and secretion of the hormone.

WHY

The Pineal.

***Balances** night and day; rest with activity.*

- Induces drowsiness and sleep at night.
- Awakening/wakefulness during daylight hours.
- Induces calm.

Also:-

- Regulates the onset of puberty.
- Seems to respond, through its neural responses, to lunar phases, determining normal 28 day menstrual cycle.

Melatonin in animals determines hibernation!

Glossary.

Capsule:…sac containing fluid.
Cerebellum:…hind brain controlling body movement & stability.
Cerebrum:…higher brain.
Connective tissue:…supports and holds specialised groups of cells together.
Corpus callosum:…mass of white nerve fibres connecting the two hemispheres of the brain.
Fornix:...arch.
Hypothalamus:…control/relay centre for neural messages to and from the body and the endocrine system/cerebrum. (some seratonin also found here.)
Inhibitory:…something that stops/prevents.
Lunar Phases:…changes of the moon.
Masses:…groups of cells for a particular function.
Meninges:…semi-transparent membranes or thin skins covering the brain.
Neuroglia:…(*Neuro* = nerve..*glia* = glue) connective nervous tissue that surrounds & supports nerve endings (neurones) with various functions.
Neurotransmitter:…chemical substance released by neuron to communicate with the next one.
Optic Nerve:…large nerve from eye to brain.
Sagittal:…side view.
Thalamus:…area of grey matter (nerve cells) under brain for senses/emotions/arousal. (some seratonin also found here.)
Ventricle:…chamber.

'SAD' Seasonal Affective Disorder is newly-identified,. This is a type of depression that occurs during dark winter months.
Light sources simulating sunlight is used as the treatment.
Can be used for jet-lag after travel through several time zones.

******

Associated Energy Centre for The Pineal Gland.

The Pineal gland is anatomically the highest so it is served and affected by the highest energy centre, known as the **Crown** chakra[1]. This is the seat of **Higher Thought**, or **Spirituality**. The condition of its circulating energy influences the whole cerebral cortex or upper brain where we think and reason.

7th The Crown Chakra

Spiritual aspiration
Positive reasoning
Clarity of thought
Self value/appraisal
Self-discipline
Evaluating concept of self in context with others
Comprehension of surroundings
Evaluation of activities/time values

All these come from our conscious cerebral activity or the intellect, ie: the whole area of the brain that lies directly above the Pineal.

Positive energy sources that energize this chakra.

- **Physical**: …….Normal balanced function of the gland.
  Positive cerebral activity and responses as per above.
- **Metaphysical**: **The Higher Self/Thought/Spirituality**.

Emotional concepts and ideas formed from the *function* of the Pineal gland are produced in the higher brain from the circumstances or disruption of normal pattern of 'production' or 'inhibition' of melatonin and its role in night/day; reproduction/puberty and the levels of seratonin.

Here we will look at this connection and see what negative thinking and memories that are related to the pineal function, (both *conscious* and *subconscious*) enter the energy of this organ. They therefore cloud and block the circulation in the **Crown** centre. This impairs the flow that is needed for clear thinking and self value.

WHAT

The consequence of imbalance and blockage in this energy centre are:
Confusion, doubt and despair.

[1] *See* **Section 2,** The Energy Centres for further information on chakras.

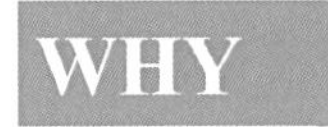

WHY

Sources of negative energy. 1)

Internal Physical.

- Broken sleep; patterns set up from past or present circumstances.
- Prolonged wakefulness, frequent disturbances and/or agitation.
- Rising for work in the dark.
- Long working hours in artificial light.
- Unusual circumstances of prolonged adrenalin output.
- Daytime working in windowless areas with artificial light.

Internal Emotional.

Associations/memories built up over time.
Self; emotionally-based associations from differing levels of **darkness,** both *conscious* and *subconscious.*

- Fear of the dark.
- Its associations; *Danger, Loneliness, Isolation, Abandonment etc.*
- Insecurity in poor lighting.

Associated negative reactions from Work and/or Sexual activity.

- Resentment, Anger, Distress.
- Anxiety, non-fulfilment, frustration.
- Insecurities in night-time social/sexual activities.

Sources of negative energy. 2)

There are also external sources which can and do create *conscious* and *subconscious* negative responses in the individual to related pineal activity in above situations.

External Physical.

- The sensory organs; *sight sound, smell* & their memory associations.
- Adverse surroundings.
- Stressors from eg: chronic illness, prolonged emotional ordeals.

External Emotional.

Sexual partners/family/friends/associates/colleagues.

- Affected by their own *internal* associations and emotional reactions causing responses or reaction of negativity in us.
- Chain-reaction from our own negativity tied in to negative memories and associations.

Our work and our gender identity and activities make up a large part of our lives. The interplay of people and events and feelings both *conscious* and *subconscious* that arise from these situations influence and affect our thinking and emotions. (*See **Sect. 3***)

It is possible now to see the *source* of aspects of our negative thinking that block the circulation of energy of the **Crown** chakra. This causes the varying degrees of confusion, doubts and despair that colour so much of our personal and working lives. Thus imbalance will impair the effects of melatonin and seratonin that are needed to balance our moods and induce rest and calm to help our thinking.

HOW

Any level of blockage **prevents** and/or **impairs** the essentials we all need for a balanced way of life so that it is in *our* control. (ergo *clear thinking*, *decision-making*, *positive self-evaluation* plus *gender outlook*, *time evaluation* and *self-discipline.*)
(When these aspects become very difficult for people, they are then Clinically Depressed. They become unable to get on with even everyday activities and decisions and therefore feel out of control. This sense of lack of control then undermines them further.)

When confused or in despair we naturally run our hands through our hair or clutch at it. **a**) indicates site of blockage; **b**) the natural instinct to clear it. These 'actions' are used in Indian Head massage for clearing the crown chakra.

PHYSICAL CONSEQUENCE.

for eg:

- headaches
- lack of motivation
- generally feeling unwell.
- general listlessness.

local conditions or illnesses, (will often linger or be recurring).

Stronger or serious deep issues from these aspects, would manifest problems in those areas of the body to where the heavier, deep subconscious negativity has gravitated to the lower chakras.

A negative connection will therefore be held between the Pineal, the **Crown** chakra and the other organs or their associated chakras. Consequently any physical manifestations anywhere else in the body that are *accompanied* by any degree of confusion, doubt and despair would indicate that:-

Healing/releasing is needed in the **Pineal** area as well as the site of the condition or illness to give the greatest effect. Attention focused on the **Crown** chakra therefore can greatly enhance the treatment being given.

If possible consider/encourage improving sleep-patterns with, for example relaxing techniques, small comfort bedtime rituals (not food!), refraining from late-night eating and drinking where possible especially on workdays or before important events.

Strategies for dealing effectively with emotional ties are explored in **Chapter 21.** These clear trapped negativity in the organs and centres and greatly improve your vitality.

All positive thinking is good, but some people can't find or can't accept a positive aspect to the problems they have..Even to raise them, or wish to reveal them is difficult, so if possible consider/suggest that as negative thoughts come up use/try:-

'Positive Distraction Thinking'.
Thinking of or doing something pleasurable or interesting quickly instead to boost the positive energy to stop the negative energy building up.

WHAT

The **Crown** chakra cannot absorb all the negativity that can be created from this region. Although the source of the energy is from the Pineal, it is mainly the negative ***thoughts*** and ***ideas*** from the cerebral activity and aspects that will collect and slow down or block the circulating energy in this seat of **Higher Thought** or **Spirituality**. The **heavier** energy will descend but will leave an associated residue of that negativity behind.

The various intensities of Pineal negative emotional energy will **gravitate** to the other chakras.

Different aspects will occupy *different* chakras.

Just as the anatomical structures are inter-related and therefore *connected*, so are the energy centres. Thus other areas of the body are affected *from* the initial source.

- Hopelessness/inability to see ahead will block the **BROW** chakra.
- Tension from unspoken sexual distress/frustration will descend to **THROAT** chakra.
- Sadness/self-pity/grief will descend to the **HEART** chakra.
- Anxiety/thwarted will/negative ego will descend to the **SOLAR PLEXUS** chakra.
- Sexual negativity will descend to the **SACRAL** chakra.
- Fear/anger/hatred, etc. will descend to the **ROOT** chakra.

Thus the whole body is affected and involved in the effects of negative energy making us feel tired and out of sorts, both mentally and physically in a non-specific way, quite apart from inhibiting the body's abilities to heal the illnesses and conditions that beset us. When you feel you aren't 'right', then negative thinking and issues are being held in the system. Your body is asking you to think things through.

Understanding the reasons for low energy and problems that can and do occur helps us to deal with them. Not knowing what could be wrong increases negativity. Knowing and acknowledging are the first steps that reduce negative thinking so that a positive attitude enables us to begin to improve our energy.

Physical conditions and illnesses in this area will naturally attract the emotional energy related to specific issues from the function of the Pineal. This will slow up or even hold up the healing process. Clearing and ridding yourself of these related issues through releasing techniques, (*See* **Chapter 21**) will alleviate the condition considerably.

Even just releasing the minor negativity of feeling miserable about being unwell or ill, will speed recovery. In using the techniques in Chapter 21 you will be surprised to find how much they are part of how you feel.

All work on the energy system to restore the flow will aid any healing process and there are several therapies designed for this too. All will also aid healthy and balanced hormonal and chakra activity. This will help the body make better use of any medication or conventional treatment as well.

Anatomically this area balances dark and light - ie: our physical timeline.
Metaphysically, higher thought or spirituality - ie: enlightenment, balances dark negative moods/emotions.

My Personal Notes

My Personal Notes

Chapter 3. The Pituitary Gland. (hypophysis)

This gland is known as the Master gland. It is the Director of Operations for all the other glands. The blood stream and the nervous system connect it to the rest of the endocrine system. Several things stimulate or inhibit the Pituitary gland: high or low levels of hormones released into the blood at need, chemical variations that require hormonal adjustment and neural messages informing of necessity for fine-tuning of cellular activity. The Pituitary then sends out what is needed from its own hormones, inhibits them or triggers the other glands to specific activity to keep a perfect and constant balance throughout the whole body.

It is ideally situated near the Command Centre in the brain, protected by both the surrounding cushion of the brain itself, (*See* **Fig:3.** p11) the little bony cup it sits in and the hard shell of the skull. All this indicates how vital a structure this is.

We will look at it in the context of its surroundings and activities to give a clear picture of this amazing gland.

WHAT

Two lobes, anterior (front) & posterior (back).

The two lobes of this *pea-sized* gland are also in the third ventricle, directly in line with the eye and adjacent to the fold of the cerebellum, tucked protectively into a bony depression known as the pituitary fossa. (the *sella turcica)*

These lobes hang from the oval masses of the Thalamus by a stalk-like structure. This is the *infundibulum*, (= funnel-shaped) which links the 'regions' of the Hypothalamus to the Pituitary. This physical connection creates an important inter-relationship for the body's growth, development and metabolism in these two lobes.

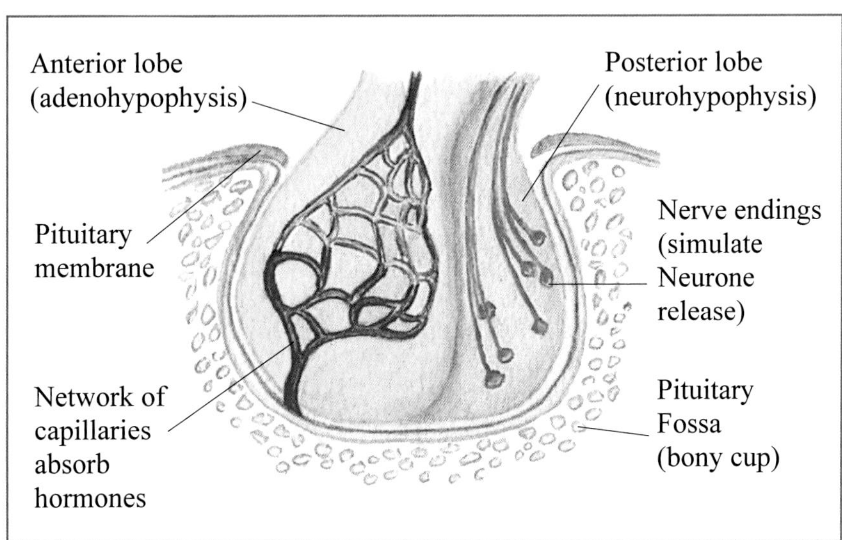

Fig 4. Both lobes of Pituitary Gland.

NB Both have *different*,
- tissue structure,
- function,
- methods of stimulation.

HOW

The Anterior Lobe. (**Adenohypophysis**)

This is **75%** of the Pituitary and is the glandular (adeno-) section.

It contains glandular epithelial cells because it is formed from the tissue of the roof of the mouth.

There are **seven** hormones produced and secreted in this lobe;
five are major **trophic** hormones.

- Controls activities of Testes/ovaries, mammaries, adrenals, thyroid, metabolism of fats/carbohydrates.
- Synthesis is stimulated via the *blood stream*, by hypothalamic hormones acting on impulses from the brain.
- It is more vascular.

Pituitary hormones that act directly on **body tissue**:-

Somatroph. (*soma* = body. *troph* = nourishment)
Produces the **H**uman **G**rowth **H**ormone, (HGH)
- controls growth in the young.
- maintains bone and muscle size and tissue repair in adulthood.
- stimulates fat and glucose metabolism.

A fat-metabolising hormone that produces ketone bodies. (fatty acids)

A blood sugar-raising principle, which has an opposite (antagonistic) action to Insulin as a *counter-balance* to maintain correct blood sugar levels.

Melanocyte-stimulating hormone, (MSH) for skin pigmentation.
Subsidiary of Corticotroph so also thought to maintain sensitivity of adrenals.

*Hyper*glycæmia, *over*-stimulation of the Islets of Langerhans (where insulin is synthesised) in the pancreas induces excess insulin production, reducing blood glucose levels. If this over-production continues, the Islets of Langerhans *fail* and Type 1 Diabetes *(Diabetes Mellitus)* results. Insulin has to be given (injected) to compensate, to regulate the glucose content of the blood, which has become artificially high because insulin production by the pancreas is now *low.* (*See also* p27)

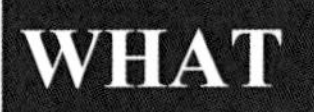

Pituitary hormones that stimulate **other** endocrine glands:-

Lactotroph. (stimulated by pregnancy**)**
Produces **Prol**actin (PRL) for milk production in the female.
During milk production, ie: **high** levels of **PRL**, fertility is reduced hormonally by withholding menstruation, ie: inhibiting.
Luteinising **H**ormone. **(LH/ovaries**). (*See* p24)

Hyper-secretion of PRL causes cessation of menstrual cycle.
In the male, it causes impotence.

Corticotroph. Produces **A**dreno**c**ortrophic **h**ormone (**ACTH**) promotes development and health of cortex (outer layer) of **Adrenal** gland and stimulates it to produce and secrete:-

a) *glucocorticoids* for utilising glucose for:-
Stimulating production of *epinephrine* (adrenalin) for everyday activities.

b) *gonadocorticoids*.
Release of androgens. ie: *testosterone*.

c) *aldosterone.*
Maintains normal blood sodium (salt) levels.
A hypertensive (raising blood pressure) when blood volume drops, (bleeding; dehydration) stimulates the kidneys to retain *sodium* and works in conjunction with:-

Anti**d**iuretic **h**ormone (**ADH** which stimulates the kidneys to retain *fluid*).
Works with epinephrine as anti-inflammatory agent in injury etc.

Hypo-secretion of glucocorticoids causes: Addison's Disease; produces mental lethargy anorexia, nausea etc.
ACTH is given very effectively.)

Thyrotroph.
Produces Thyroid-stimulating hormone. (**TSH**)
Enables **Thyroid** to secrete its hormones.

Gonadotroph.
Stimulates **Testes** and **Ovaries.**
Produces:-

1. **Follicle-stimulating hormone. (FSH)**
   This in turn stimulates:-
   - Ova production. (development of graafian follicles where ova develop)
   - Secretion of œstrogen in follicle cells in ovaries.
   - Sperm production in testes. (gonads)
2. **Luteinising hormone. (LH)**
   In conjunction with **FSH**, stimulates:-
   - Ovulation.
   - Secretion of œstrogen.
   - Formation of Corpus Luteum (ripe follicle ready for ovulation) and its secretion, progesterone.
   - Secretion of testosterone in testes.

HOW

Quick summary of main Pituitary Hormones

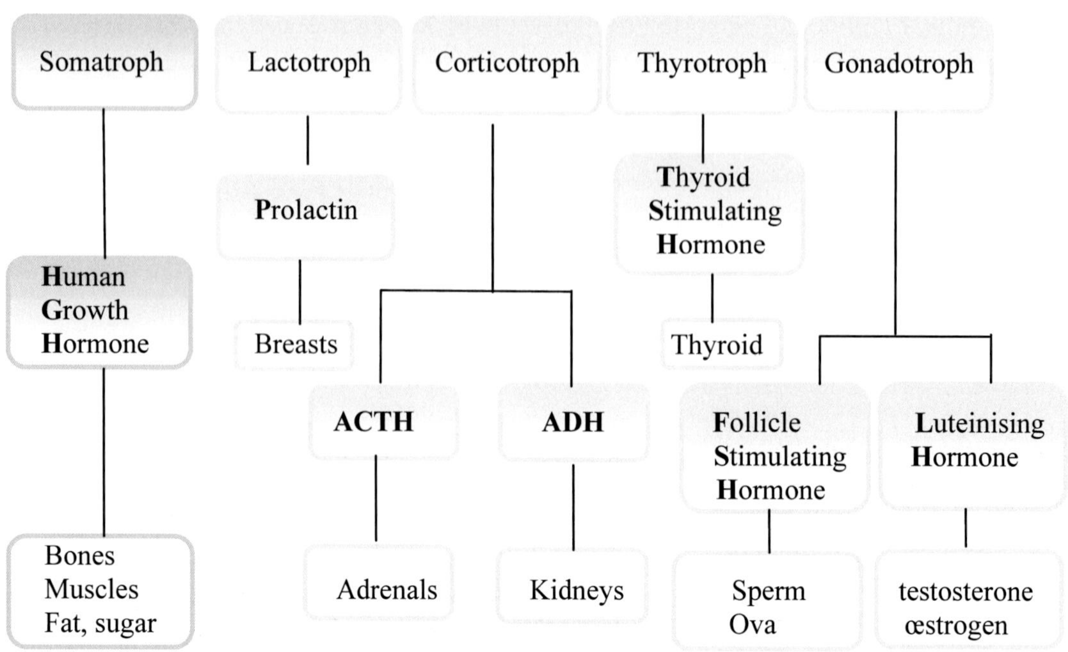

Changes/Increases in Reproductive Hormones.

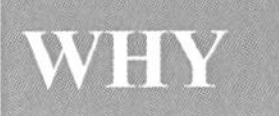

Increases in secretions of **FSH** and **LH** (Gonadotrophin)
during pre-menstruation and menstrual cycle effect changes in **blood** glucose (controlled by **ACTH**) and saline levels (controlled by Corticotrophin/aldosterone).

Negative feedback mechanism results in the Hypothalamus stimulating:-

- Hunger centre….urge for chocolate and/or food to increase glucose,
- Antidiuretic hormone **ADH**, to inhibit urine excretion, stimulating *water retention*. The combination of **ADH** and **Aldosterone** effects an increase in blood volume possibly for the expected development of the endometrial (interior) lining of the uterus, or loss in menstruation.

The blood glucose needs adjusting to accommodate the increased volume, thus the stimulation from the hypothalamus for increased sugar intake.

Increases in the system will affect the changes, the body's adjustments and time taken to correct the balance efficiently. Thus water retention and/or the sugar/food urge *can persist past the body's needs*. (as many women know!) This creates imbalance.

HOW

Imbalances in Testosterone, Progesterone and Œstrogen.

Mostly at onset of puberty.

- Later testosterone surges in males.
- Pre-ovulation, (PMT) surges.
- Menopausal fluctuations.

Symptoms

- Mood swings.
- Aggressive/emotional behaviour.
- Acne and facial eruptions.

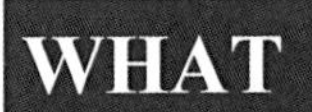

Stress syndrome.

High production of **CRH** involves the pituitary, limbic system and cerebrum. This leads to increased **ACTH**. **ADH**, and aldosterone in the blood stream. The longer it takes for the body to re-adjust, the longer the body is under stress. This can lead to a spiralling effect. (*See* Chap: 8)

Posterior Lobe. (**Neuro**hypophysis)
As the name suggests, activity in this lobe is neurological in nature.

WHY

Developed from cerebral tissue. Contains axon terminals. Hormones are not synthesised in this lobe.

Two hormones are **stored** and **released** here from its cells called **pituicytes.** These receptor cells are in the terminals of neurosecretory axons running through the infundibulum channel from the neurosecretory cells in the hypothalamus.

HOW

Stimulus for lobe's activity (storage or release) is from neurological *signals* from the hypothalamus.

Stimulus for hypothalamic neural activity is from *blood hormone and saline levels.*

WHY

The two stored hormones are:-

1) Oxytocin (OT) (*oxys* = swift. *tokos* = childbirth).

This has two targets in pregnancy.

- *Uterus*, for contractions during labour and delivery, and placental expulsion. (*See* further Hypothalamus definition below)
  Released further during suckling,
  to aid contraction of womb to normal size. (positive feedback mechanism)
- *Breasts*, for milk ejection from stimuli of suckling or the baby's cry.

A **contractor** of **smooth** muscle, this hormone also acts on:-

i) The blood vessels; to control pressure.
ii) The intestines.
iii) Gall bladder.
iv) Urinary bladder.

Necessary for the movement of their contents and expulsion of their bi-products. (*See* **ANS,** p149.)

All muscular movement ie: exercise, 'massages' blood vessels to help maintain flow and aid correct pressure. That's why exercise is good for us

2) Antidiuretic hormone. (ADH)
Antidieuresis = opposing the production of large volumes of urine.
It has two actions:-

1) Acts on the tubules of the kidney:

- Maintains correct water balance in body, by r*egulating* the flow of urine.
- It raises blood pressure in case of serious loss of blood volume (either bleeding or dehydration) by stimulating the kidneys to decrease urine excretion by returning water by osmosis to the bloodstream.

2) Acts on the blood vessels:-

- Pressor action as a vasoconstrictor. constricts capillaries and arterioles. This would prevent further blood volume loss. (This substance is often called Vassopressin.)

WHAT

Hypo-activity of, or damage to, the posterior pituitary lobe causes Diabetes *Insipidus*. (No glucose in urine) ADH production is inhibited so water balance is disrupted and severe dehydration results without hormone replacement to correct the deficiency.

*Hyper*glycæmia: high glucose levels in blood ie: Type 1 Diabetes, *Diabetes Mellitus,* (*See also* p 23) is a Pancreatic disorder, but involves the pituitary through negative feedback needed to stimulate insulin production.

Laxness (under-activity) in the smooth muscle/conditions involving the smooth muscle:

- Constipation,
- Irritable bowel syndrome,
- Varicose veins,
- Weak bladder.
- Colitis.
- Arteriosclerosis.

It is important to observe the **interplay** between these two lobes, despite their differences.

- Both deal with aspects of reproduction.
- Both have actions and interactions concerning the adrenals which involve the homeostasis of the blood.
- Both are activated by the Hypothalamus, which is in turn in constant neurological contact with the cerebral cortex.

The whole area that the Pituitary gland is specifically connected to is an extremely important centre that deals with the function of the pituitary gland. Because it is so essential, understanding it will give a broader picture of the hormonal system so I have included the vital statistics here of the connecting stalk and the particular 'regions'.

The Infundibulum.

WHAT

This is the channel connecting the two lobes of Pituitary individually to the Hypothalamus.

Internal.
Connects the **posterior** lobe to brain centre.

Carries neurosecretory axons (nerve fibres) from the secretory nerve cells in the Hypothalamus to the axon endings in this lobe of the Pituitary for hormonal activity.

External.
Connects the **anterior** lobe to brain centre.

It has a rich capillary network which branches off from the superior hypophyseal artery. This brings oxygen-rich blood to the network.
This hypophyseal portal system connects the Hypothalamus with this lobe of the Pituitary for synthesising and secreting its hormones.

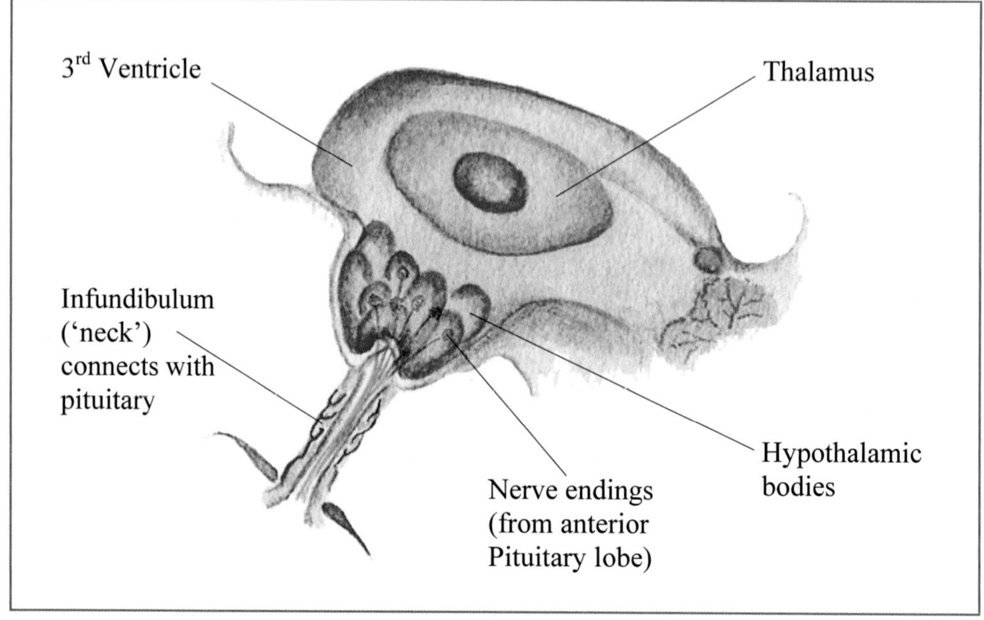

Fig:5. The Diencephalon and Infundibulum.

The Diencephalon. (= 'between' brain) (Gk. *dia* = through, *enkephalos* = brain).

WHAT

This area of the brain, tucked protectively under the cerebrum in the third ventricle, right in the centre of the brain mass, is an amazing and important area. It is the *information relay centre,* the *messenger service* and *sorting office* between the body and the brain, both conscious and unconscious, and the hormonal system, and is therefore essential to our understanding of the connections between them.

It consists of two parts with two related but separate functions.

1) The *Thalamus* (Gk; '*inner*' chamber).
Large, paired, oval mass of **nerve cells** (grey matter) under the cerebrum at either side of the third ventricle. There are several nuclei for the variety of information and tasks.

These smooth egg-shaped thalami have a thin outer covering of white matter. They act as a confluence for most **sensory impulses** before they pass out to the **cerebral cortex** where subtle and complex interpretations are made.

Joining them across the ventricle is a bridge of grey matter, the neurons of **the intermediate mass.**

HOW

This area of the brain is like a Call Centre, taking in messages and relaying them on to the relevant section of the nervous system or endocrine glands to keep everything working smoothly to balance all the functions of the body so that they help each other.

Information comes in from:-

Sensory systems……sight, smell, taste, etc, memory from Limbic system.

- Cerebral hemispheres…conscious brain.
- Cerebellum…………co-ordinates movements/muscle tone, (unconscious).
- Grey matter in the **A**utonomous (unconscious) **N**ervous **S**ystem: **S**ympathetic **N**ervous **S**ystem (wholly responsible for release of Adrenalin).
- Grey matter in **P**arasympathetic **N**ervous **S**ystem part of **ANS** in brain stem & sacral region of spinal cord.
  (conserves/restores body energy as counter-balance to adrenalin responses)
  ANS deals with all information to and from internal organs. (*See* Chap: 9)

WHY

These are all integrated and correlated here before information is sent to the relevant area of cerebral cortex where it is interpreted stored and action initiated. This is via the white matter (nerve fibres) within the body of the brain, fanning out to all areas and connecting the hemispheres with one another across the corpus callosum to make best possible use of the information received.

Here the '*higher* brain' ie: intellect/cerebral cortex **connects** with the '*lower*' brain' unconscious/midbrain.

WHERE

2) The ***Hypothalamus.***
This lies under (=hypo-) the Thalamus. The Hypothalamus actually forms part of the walls and floor of the third ventricle. It has four 'regions' clustered above the infundibulum. They each contain several hormones which are synthesised.

HOW

This section is the Sorting Office as it has its own hormones that *stimulate* and *suppress* hormonal activity. This makes the Hypothalamus a major player in the task of homeostasis.

Functions.

- Hypothalamus regulates and co-ordinates the **unconscious** functions of the body.
- Body's balancing act, thanks to its Releasing and Inhibiting hormones that are the regulating 'feedback' system vital for **homeostasis.**

Two methods of activity.
1) **Neural** information and release.

Neuro-secretary stimulation for **posterior** lobe of pituitary gland.

- Oxytocin and ADH.

For storage and release.
Passed from cells along the axons in the infundibulum to the nerve terminals in the posterior lobe.

2) **Blood stream** information and secretion.

Blood supply stimulation for **anterior** lobe of pituitary gland; 'releasing' or 'inhibiting' hormones (for all hormones) which *stimulate* or *suppress* their hormonal activity.
Secreted into its own blood supply to target cells in the lobe, (hypophyseal portal system).
for eg:

- Somatocrinin; **G**rowth **h**ormone ***r****eleasing* **h**ormone: **GHRH**.
- Somatostatin **G H** *inhibiting* **h**ormone; **GHIH** etc.

Activated by **internal** organs; *Initiation and Response is immediate.*
from:-

- osmotic pressure.
- blood temperature and volume.
- blood glucose and saline levels.
- hormonal concentration levels.

WHAT

Control and integration of neural activity from **ANS** (unconscious brain) for:-

Contraction of smooth muscle of **digestive** and **urinary** tracts.
Regulating **heart beat** and controlling contraction of Cardiac muscle
Regulating, through specialised centres:

- **body temperature**.
- fluid levels.
- **hunger** (from blood sugar levels).
- **thirst** (from blood salt levels).

Synthesis of hormones.
Maintaining **waking** and **sleep** patterns.

N.B. Those autonomous bodily functions highlighted in **bold** involve the 'conscious' brain.
They can be changed by the conscious brain as a reaction to ***emotional*** *thinking.*

HOW

Sensory receptors in the Hypothalamus are connected to the cerebral cortex via the Thalamus. They are **stimulated by**:-

- Sensory systems……sight, smell, taste, hearing etc,…
- Limbic system. ie: 'the Emotional brain',……………...
- Reticular activating system (relay network in the brainstem.)
- Cerebral cortex.
- Thalamus.

The close integration of the nervous and endocrine systems in the Hypothalamus is the important connection here for all aspects of healing.

Thus thinking' *and* hypothalamic hormonal responses both come from external stimuli.

It is this 'higher' brain influence,
ie: 'mind over matter' that accounts for:-

- Hypochondria.
- Psychosomatic symptoms.

But also,

- Self-healing.
- Positive thinking effects.

WHAT

The hypothalamus is also the centre for **feelings of rage** and **aggression.** As well as receiving sensory stimuli and cerebral interpretation, hypothalamic activity closely inter-relates with both hormonal glands dealing with:-

- reproduction/sexuality (pituitary).
- the stress control system and 'flight or fight' response. (adrenals)
- release of gonadocorticoids and androgens. (adrenals)

(Originally geared for survival, man's sophisticated thinking, society and its value systems have taken these functions into very broad realms of behaviour and response.)

The anatomical connection in this region here between the sex-related hormones system, rage and aggression and the 'emotional' brain (the Limbic) is an important one.

WHY

The **balancing** and **harmonising** of its intricate hormonal activities for the whole body are the fundamental and essential functions of the Diencephalon.

Balance and **harmony** for the whole body are also the fundamental and essential concepts in true healing.

Glossary.

CRH:…**C**orticotrophin **R**eleasing **H**ormone.

Diabetes:…[GK. for '*pass through*'] collective name for symptoms from high blood sugar levels.

Grey matter:…nerve cells where messages are received, interpreted and responses transmitted.

Hyper-…above …more than.

Hypo-….under …less than.

Hypochondria:…intense chronic interest in one's health/being convinced of suffering from ill-health.

Hypophysis:…below body of brain.

Nocturnal eneursis:…bed-wetting.

Osmosis:…fluid/molecules can pass through membrane one way but not back again.

Ovum:…egg…plural; **ova**.

Psychosomatic:…symptoms caused or made worse by emotional belief in them.

Retention:…holding back.

Reticular activating system:…relay network in brainstem for maintaining consciousness.

White matter:…fibres carrying messages in electrical impulses to and from brain and body.

CRH Corticotropin **r**eleasing **h**ormone stimulates secretion of both corticotropin (saline levels) & MSH melanocyte stimulating hormone for skin pigmentation.

******

The Interbrain or 'Emotional Brain'.

This area we will look at now is known as the Limbic system. It is connected via the physical links of neurological brain tissue to the Pineal and the Pituitary so it will be helpful to you to have some idea about this fascinating area of the brain that balances the emotions, wants and needs of the body for survival.

WHY

Because emotions are the cause of positive and negative thinking and the energy produced affects both our mental and physical energy, exploring the connections in the brain where emotions originate will be immensely helpful. Emotions have a physical origin; they are not just formless feelings that we just happen to have. They are an essential part of survival. *They develop our memories*. They also have associations to learn from for that purpose. This enables us to '*experience*' our life as well as survive because man can consciously *recall* memories. Emotions arise subconsciously from our memories and associations and have a direct bearing on behaviour and our relationships.

WHAT

A 'border' or ring of structures composed of grey matter, surrounds this vital region. It runs from the inner rim of the cerebrum along the corpus callosum that links the two hemispheres, to the floor of the 3rd ventricle, and encircles the brain stem directly below it. Convolutions (gyri) of the brain, fold between the structures. These portions of the cerebrum inter-relate with the several structures.

The Limbic System *(limbus* = border).

The Interbrain and sometimes called the '*emotional*' brain.
This complex area is highly subtle. It contrives to balance the *extremes* of emotion, between fear/terror and desire/ecstasy.
(It is still not well understood.)
The main function is **behaviour** for **survival.**

Its major component is the hippocampus (= 'seahorse') enfolded by the cerebral dentate gyrus. Nerve cell masses are linked to the cerebrum through a vast network of connective axons: bundles of myelinated (sheathed) fibres. These not only inform the limbic system from *sensory/motor impulses* but also carry information back, which initiates *physical reactions*, ie: shivering/trembling, sweating/flushing/blushing, etc . *Seratonin* counter-acts these responses. (*See* Pineal/Adrenals)
These are all defence responses to initiate defensive physical behaviour....all are allied to the emotions fear and anxiety made complex in sophisticated man. However they also relate to desire and ecstasy - but these are still to do with survival of the species.

The Limbic structures are closely connected into this whole communications area.

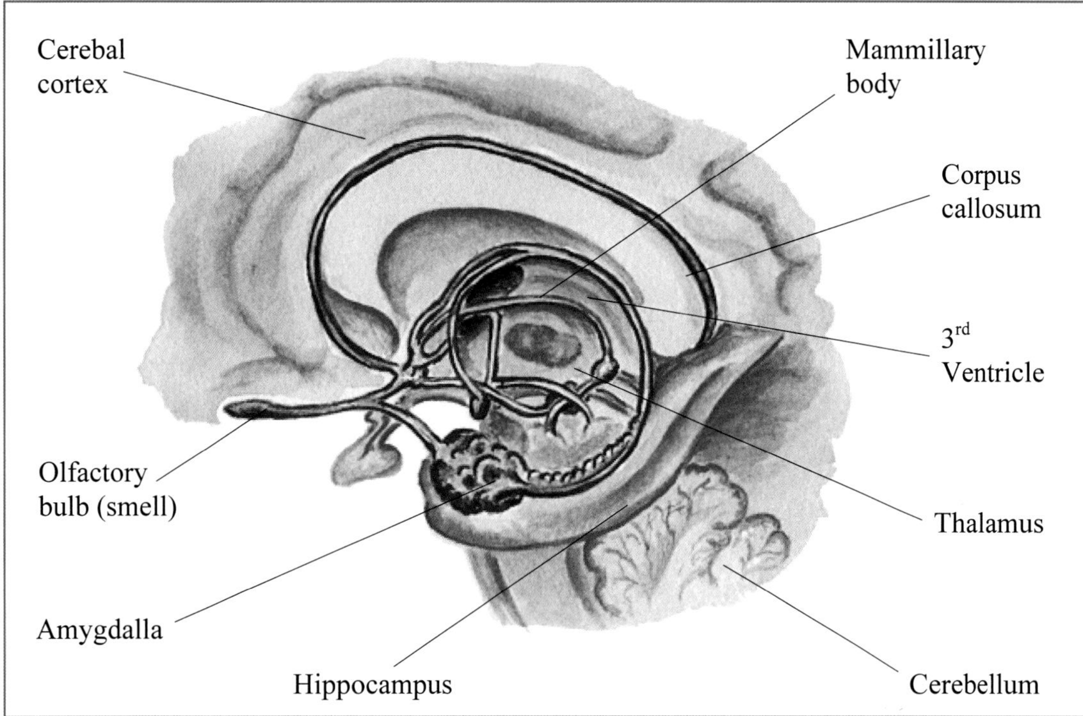

Fig:6. The Limbic system.

The combined activity of the limbic system is
Storage and Retrieval of memory.
Responses are from neural connection to the hypothalamus and other *autonomic* centres.

- The stronger the emotional link, the clearer and more profound is the memory.
- Experience is also an important factor.

WHY

The integrated Limbic system as a whole:

Contains centres for pleasure and pain, both have *neurological* and *emotional* links to memory. This includes the *wide variety* of grades of:-

- Fear, anger, rage, sorrow, sexual feelings, docility, affection.

Controls *in*voluntary aspects of behaviour/response.

Connected to the initial *subconscious* response to people and situations.

- These factors are all essential for **relationships:** *personal, social* and *working*.

HOW

Directly linked into the limbic system are the olfactory lobes, containing sensory receptors from the nose. Odours are strongly evocative.
Primitively Scent can indicate danger or recognition of compatibility/sexual readiness etc.; It is also part of sexual attraction.

All are essential and for the purpose of **survival**. We are less primitive now but body fragrance and our perfumes are our sexual nosegay, and we learn the dangerous smells through experience. These all form essential memories and associations for us.

The structures that comprise the Limbic system are physically linked into one circular structure creating an enclosed 'island'. This *surrounds* and is *in contact with,* the gyri, connective axons, grey matter and endocrine glands of this area of the brain. This is where the 'higher' brain connects and inter-links with the 'between' brain, midbrain, interbrain and brainstem.

> This relationship between the 'conscious' and the 'unconscious' brain, should be of note and significance to all aspects of healing. (*See* Chap: 16)

This system, though not fully understood, adds to the enrichment of our conscious lives and our *subconscious social connections with each other.* (*See* ***Section 3***)

Physical and **psychological** (emotional) trauma can affect this area, inducing:-

> • Loss of short and long term memory: temporary and permanent.
> • Acute and Chronic aggressive and/or anti-social behaviour.
>
> These play an essential part in all social communication and relationships.
> *The potential for negativity is high.*
>
> • From the person.
> • From the variety of responses from individuals and society.

Because the stronger the emotional experience is to the memory, the more influence that memory has on our subconscious vibrational connection with people. (*See* ***Section 3***)
Rage and aggression and other effects of fear through subconscious expectation can come to the surface unexpectedly if an associated memory, however small, triggers it off. Clearing these emotional links therefore, is important. They can be reasoned into submission but remain in the brain's archives unless released. (*See* Chap: 16)

Before we move on to the energy centre associated with this area it would be helpful to take a brief look at the upper brain itself. It lies between the two energy centres the **crown** and **brow** chakras after all so will be subject to the energy from both.

The Cerebrum. (seat of the intellect; Central Nervous System.)

Having looked at the neurological connections in the Diencephalon between the pituitary and the 'emotional' brain or Limbic system, and the upper brain, it would be helpful to look at the main anatomy of the Cerebrum that interprets all those neurological signals. After all, the upper brain is where evaluation of life's experiences is made, memories formed and, as a natural consequence, our *emotional connections* develop.

It is a complex organ but we can take a brief look at the specialisms within this incredible structure to get some idea of its basic workings.

WHAT

The major part of the brain.

The Cerebrum......... (the forebrain)

- Two hemispheres divided by a deep central groove, known as a fissure. (the sagittal fissure)
- The hemispheres control opposite sides of the body.
- The surface of this layer is greatly increased by many folds called convolutions or gyri (singular = gyrus): the greater the area, the higher the intelligence....(man has the most convolutions).
- The shallow grooves between are called sulci, deep grooves are called fissures.
- Each hemisphere is sub-divided into **lobes** or areas. These correspond with the cranial bones that cover them.

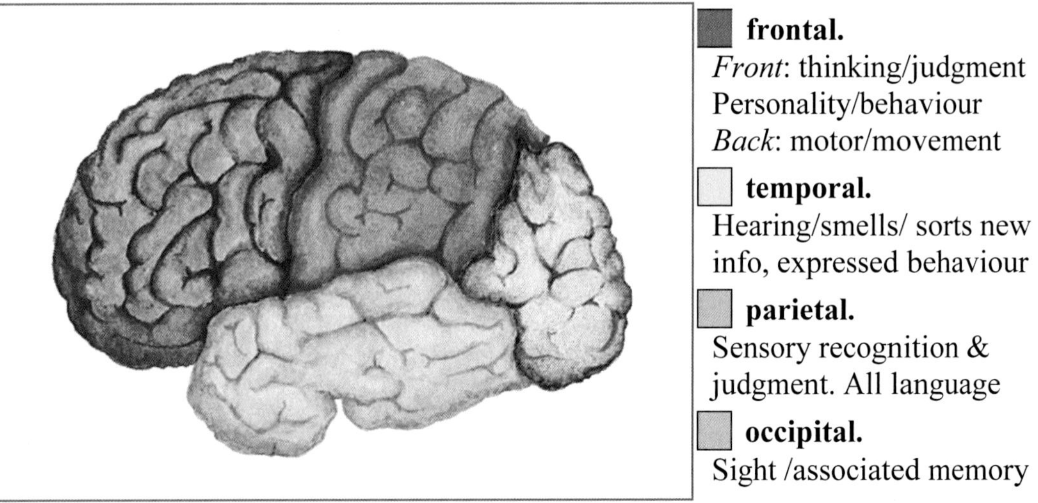

Fig:7. The main lobes. (*See* p 42)

The main component is the neurone, the nervous tissue of the brain. (*See* **Fig:2.** p10)

The cerebrum has two layers:-

The first layer is a thin layer of **grey** matter only 2 - 4 mms thick made up of the nerve **cells**, (neurons) the neucleated part of the neurone.

This is where the brain *receives* information and then *transmits* directions/instructions to the body via the neurones. *Everything* is stored, analysed and responded to. Here we do our thinking, analysing, *interpreting* and decision-making from the information and memories the brain *gathers* and *stores* to work from.

HOW

1) The cerebral cortex.

Six layers composed of:-
- **Cerebral neurons**: 'excitable' nerve cells, ie: take electrical charge. (**nerve cells** with their **axon terminals** and **dendrites)**.
- bundles of *un*myelinated axons.
- **neuroglia.**

Neuroglia (*Gk..neuro..*nerve..*glia..*glue) surrounds and supports these essential neurons. It is an amazing highly active mass of tissue that **connects**, **nourishes** and **protects** the nervous tissue so is worth understanding.

Neuroglia.

- Smaller than neurons; known as glial cells: several types.
- *Don't* take electrical charge.
- Sub-divide, therefore *can increase and replace themselves*.
- Support and connect neurons, which are embedded in them.
- Transport neurons in brain development.
- Link neurons to blood vessels for nutrients and taking away waste.
- Provide a selective filter for substances entering brain cells: known as the Blood-Brain Barrier. (*See* later, circulatory system.)
- Help in the production of cerebro-spinal fluid.
- Produce myelin sheath for nerve fibres.
- Nourish neurotransmitters.
- Balance chemical components of ions. (*See* ions below.)
- Migrate to site of injury to:-

a) replace tissue with rapid subdivision.
b) engulf and destroy dead cells and microbes.

Because they *sub-divide* neuroglia develops into a tumour, *not* neural tissue

The 2nd layer of the cerebrum contains the *lines of communication* along the nerve **fibres**. These connect hemispheres with one another and Cerebrum with **A**utonomous **N**ervous **S**ystem.

2) White matter…nerve **fibres.**

Masses of **axons.**

Carry the impulses to and from grey matter, forming *pathways*.

These have a protective **white** fatty, insulating **myelin sheath.**

- Forms small oblongs with a tiny gap between. (nodes of Ranvier)
- Gaps create the *propulsion* and *speed* of the electrical impulses known as Saltatory conduction. (saltare = to leap)
- Myalin acts as insulator to prevent impulses filtering into other tissues/organs.

If just the axon or dendrites are damaged or cut they can grow again from the axon hillock. In this way the nerve fibres can make recovery from injury and surgery.

The nerve pathways become stronger, the more they are used to carry messages.

WHAT

The two hemispheres of the brain control opposite sides of the body and have different functions.

Although the hemispheres have different specialisations, they *share* learning and memory.
Connected by the commissural fibres in the Corpus callosum which keep the two hemispheres in constant communication.

Connector fibres link hemisphere to hemisphere and nerve centre to nerve centre. This keeps the entire Central Nervous System in constant contact.

HOW

Projection fibres: The *corona radiata*. Fans and radiates from the brain stem out to the full cerebral cortex and back down to spinal cord.

Association fibres: Looping strands link different centres in the gyri of cerebral cortex in the *same* hemisphere.

Commissural fibres: These fibres cross laterally from one hemisphere to the other for constant communication and sharing of information between the two through the *Corpus callosum*.

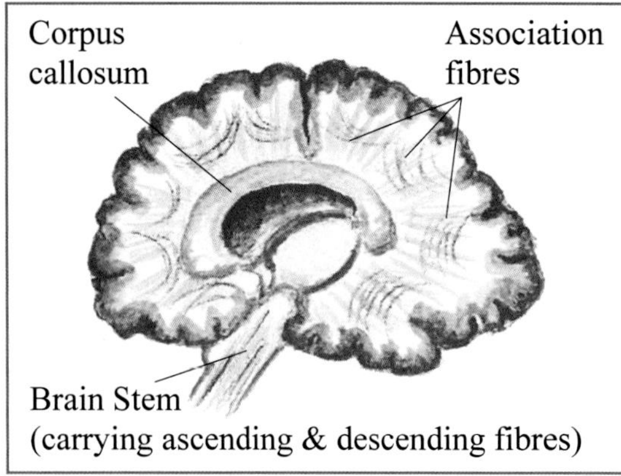

Fig:8.1. Connecting fibres.

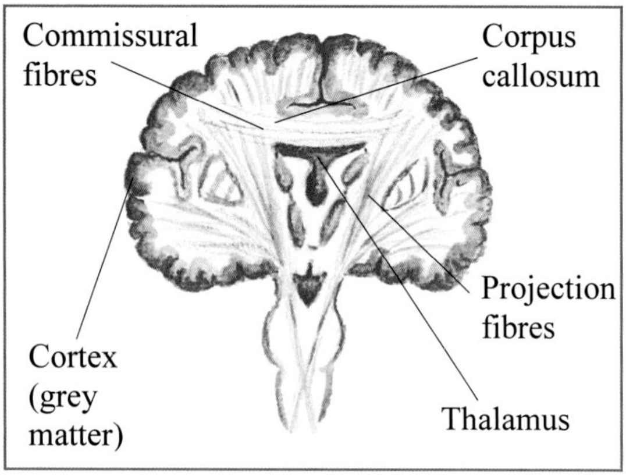

Commissural fibres
Corpus callosum
Projection fibres
Cortex (grey matter)
Thalamus

Fig:8.2. Corona radiata.

WHY

In the *female* brain, the splenium (bulge at back of C. Callosum.) is larger and more bulbous. This is because there are more fibres linking the posterior part of the brain (occipital to parietal). These *increase* the *inter-hemispheric* integration of *information.*

This probably developed from the original need for *multi-tasking* in motherhood to raise and care for several children *at the same time* and the *variety* of domestic skills.

In the *male* brain, *visual spatial skills* are *more* specialised.

This developed from the original specialised *hunting* skills.
Efficient *weapon* and *killing* skills were needed for *food/protection.*

Specialization of Hemispheres.

Left hemisphere: controls *right* side of body

Logical side/symbols. 1 dimension.

- Reasoning.
- Analytical thinking.
- Spoken and written language.
- Using and understanding sign language.
- Numeracy.
- Scientific skills/aptitude.

Right hemisphere: controls *left* side of body

Creative side/pattern/space/abstracts.

- Musical and artistic awareness.
- 3 dimensional awareness, (spatial, shape/pattern).
- Insight; shaping ideas/prompt grasp of things that relate. (Cross-referencing)
- Clearer perception of non-speech sounds.
- Better tactile perception.
- Creates mental images from sight, sound, touch, taste, and smell for comparisons & evaluation; (mind's eye).
- Imagination; inventiveness.

Usually one hemisphere is more developed neurologically, (stronger nerve pathways established) ie: more dominant, than the other. Thus we have Right handed and Left-handed people. However the close interaction and connectedness between ensures that access to all areas occurs as needed/required as determined by that dominance, sharing information and skills and expanding the brain's comprehension and interpretation.

Functions within Cerebral cortex.
In order to deal with the mass of information coming in and instructions going out of the cortex, specialised centres have developed in the lobes of the brain. These are:-
Nerve centres,.....**groups** of the **same** type of nerve cell, such as:

- *Motor;* voluntary muscular system.
- *Sensory;* skin, muscles, bones, joints.
- *Special senses;* sight, hearing, smell, taste, touch.
- *Higher mental capacity;* consciousness, intelligence, higher thought, reasoning, decision-making, memory, creativity, imagination etc.

WHY

All primary nerve centres have secondary 'association areas' alongside them. These are a specialised memory area so that the brain can readily repeat and recall all the motor and sensory things it has learned, specifically to do with each centre. They are the recognition areas from all past experiences. Interpretation is linked to the *emotions* that we associate with these memories from the activities in the Limbic system. They form part of our pre-conceptions and assumptions about new experiences and are coloured by both positive and negative thoughts and ideas as part of our learning process and decision-making. Memory, interpretation and emotions all personal to the individual, are largely unquantifiable therefore metaphysical. Yet here we can see how they originate in physical areas of the brain.

Centres in *frontal* lobe:

- Primary **Motor**.
- Secondary: **Association area**; comprehension, interpretation.
- Eyes, (eg: scanning,) head.
- Broca's area; thoughts into Speech.
- Speech; tongue, larynx, pharynx, mouth, co-ordinating breathing.

Centres in *temporal* lobe:

- Primary **Hearing**,
- Wernicke's area. **Association area**: memory, comprehension and interpretation of auditory speech, words into thoughts. Evaluation/differentiation between music, sounds, speech.
- Smell.

Centres in *parietal* lobe:

- Primary **Sensory**/body/speech/taste.
- Secondary **Association area** for sensory information ie: body position, pressure, temperature, shape, texture, relationship to other objects etc from *sensations/* perception.
  Memory storage: comparison and evaluation.
  Comprehension: interpretation.
- Gnostic area; (Gk. *gnosis* = knowledge) *integrated* with all other areas for memory, reasoning, emotions, personality traits, will, judgment and intelligence.

Centres in o*ccipital* lobe:

- Primary **Sight**. NB back of the head; far from eyes at front.
- Secondary **Association area**; visual memory storage, Comprehension, Comparison and Evaluation, Interpretation.

The **fifth** lobe of the brain is hidden. It is the Insula; also called the island of Reil.

- It lies deep in the lateral cerebral fissure, above the basal ganglia.
- Functions are largely unknown.
- Interprets signals from abdominal organs: salivation; possibly interprets taste.

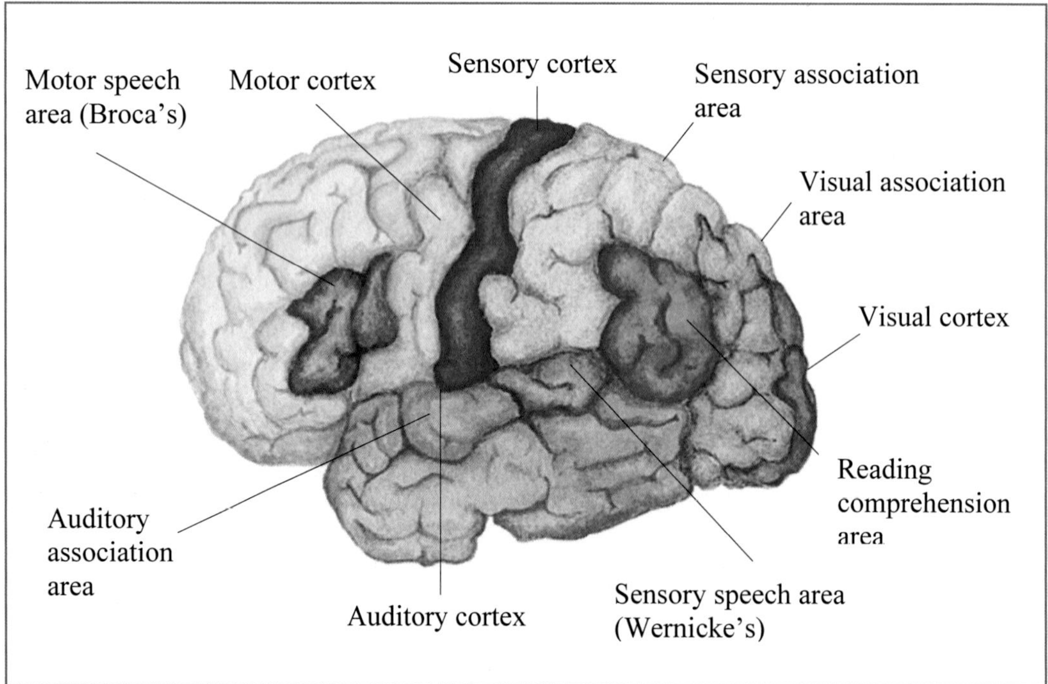

Fig:9. Centres of the brain. NB the size of the association or memory areas.

Having looked at the basic anatomy and functions of the cerebrum it's possible now to see what is involved in the thinking and memories that involve our emotions. The head chakras of **Crown** and **Brow** naturally cover this area. Thus it is easy to see why any emotional and negative shadows or blockage trapped here will impair one's thinking, evaluation and interpretation to cause confusion, doubt and poor judgment as shown in the chapters on these two energy centres.

Although medical conditions are not part of the brief of this book and therapists and healers do not diagnose medically, it might be helpful to know briefly of a few conditions as they are quite well-known.

HOW

CVA. Or Cerebro-Vascular Accident. (Stroke)

- Hæmorrhage (=bleeding) into the brain tissue from ruptured vessel, (often involves Broca's area (thoughts into speech) in the frontal lobe)

Cerebral Embolism. (= blockage: formed from blood clot/fat/air bubble) in a blood vessel preventing blood flow to area of brain.

- Damage is caused by lack of oxygen to brain cells.
- Blood clots are broken down and re-absorbed by white blood cells. (The size of the clot, re-absorption quality/abilities, will vary the recovery rate.)

Multiple sclerosis.

- Patchy degeneration of myelin sheath. Scarring (scleroses = scars) occurs.
- Breaks up the pathway for electrical charge and makes it intermittent, therefore inefficient. Poor muscle control results.
- Periods of remission (= no symptoms) occur while the degenerative process stops and the body adapts. The periods vary and can last for several years. They are followed by renewed attacks on the myalin sheath and more scarring occurs. These hardened sclerotic areas gradually increase; thus the disease is progressive.

Tumours.

It is only the glial cells in the brain, having the capacity to subdivide, that can develop into brain tumours. It is abnormalities of *cell-division* that lead to such growths; both benign, and malignant, ie: carcinoma (cancer). Most tumours of the nervous system originate in glial cells.

Benign tumours develop in a capsule, so are contained. Cancerous growths are invasive of other tissue, thus are malignant, and more harmful and difficult to deal with surgically.

NB As can be appreciated, the state of general health and mental well-being of the individual will influence the level of severity, progress, regenerative abilities and state of recovery of any condition. This also accounts for the differences and range within the signs and symptoms experienced by individuals with the same condition.

******

Glossary.

Autonomous **N**ervous **S**ystem:....deals with all spontaneous and unconscious activity eg: internal organs etc.

Axon terminals:...axons end in little branches; each end in a minute bulb, a *synaptic knob*. These terminals (ends) store neurotransmitters.

Axon:...fibre that carries information *to* and *from* the nerve cell. (*white* matter)

Cerebral:...to do with the Cerebrum.

Dendrites: (*dendro* = tree) Many-branched filaments extending from nerve cell body linking neurones to one another.

There is a tiny *gap* (*synapse)* between the endings of neighbouring dendrites. Electrical charge from neural activity jumps this gap to connect neurones to pass on the information they carry.

Diagnose:...from Gk...*Dia* = from...*gnosis* = knowledge.

Nerve:...Bundles of axons.

Neucleated:...containing the neucleus.

Nucleus:...living part of cell where cell activity takes place.

Neuron:...nerve cell **body**; does not sub-divide. (*grey* matter)

3 parts:-

- Nucleus and proteins for growth/function; renewal of damaged axons and dendrites.
- **Axon hillock**. Tapered portion which develops a thread-like process, called:
- The **initial segment**; (*grey* matter) from which axon grows.

Neurone:...complete nerve cell body plus its axon and dendrites.

Neurone *sending* impulse = presynaptic neurone. (pre- = before)
Neurone *receiving* impulse = postsynaptic neurone. (post- = after)
Grouped knots of these neurones are called **Ganglia**. *(ganglion* = knot) (*See* basal ganglia)

Neurotransmitter:...changes the *electrical* impulse into a *chemical* one and allows it to jump the *synaptic cleft*, and so transfer the information to the neuron.

These are released at the synapse, where the axons connect at the receptor sites on the neuron. These are *input* endings in the neurons. This is the *fast* axonal transport system (along mylinated fibres).
Synapse = break in the action of the impulse.
Synaptic cleft. The fluid-filled space that the break occurs in.

This is essential for *co-ordinating* homeostasis, by maintaining a constant flow of information and negative feedback mechanism.

Nerve Pathways:....Essential that these are strongly established. Sufficient time for crawling is needed for this to occur. This establishes the dominance of one hemisphere by age 5, so that the **ear, eye, hand** and **foot** are dominant on either the left *or* right.
This ensures good *motor skills*. Crawling is therefore essential and should not be shortened, discouraged or inhibited by artificial means, especially for long periods in waking hours.

Seratonin:...neuro-transmitter that controls mood, induces calm.

Sign:...evidence that can be seen, eg: swelling, rash etc.

Symptom:...change in body's function that indicates illness, eg: vomiting, sweating etc.

Vascular:...to do with blood vessels.

Associated Energy Centre for The Pituitary Gland.

The Pituitary gland is anatomically behind the eyes so it is served and affected by its energy centre, the **Brow** chakra. This is the seat of **Intuition**, **Sensitivity** and **Awareness.**

6th The Brow Chakra.
Seat of the **feminine principle.**
(feminine principle/element for both genders)

Intuition.
Instinctive discernment/appraisal.
Sensitivity to others/environment.
Awareness of 'place of 'being'/inhabiting.
Sensitivity to nature/earth/skies.
Seat of psychic abilities.

The **Brow** chakra is also known as the **Third Eye**. It intuits, 'sees' that further dimension to ordinary thinking. (Also called the Ajner; Sanskrit for Third Eye)

Positive energy sources that energize this chakra.

- **Physical**:........Normal balanced function of gland.
  Energy from nature's life force; the human perceptions of the natural world (beauty, joy, fertility etc)/all positive cerebral activity.
- **Metaphysical**: **Higher Self/Thought/Spirituality/Loving, lovingness within.**
  It is the most developed in psychics.

Instinct was our guide to the physical world until, as homo sapiens, we began to develop the intellect and intuition. The reasoning power of the intellect can and will over-ride our instincts and intuition, but these are our *primary* source of information for survival and need to be valued. Perception, discernment and interpretation are needed for cerebral activity, for ourselves, situations, perception of others and our surroundings.

Keeping the energy centre clear, allows a free flow of positive energy to energise it and also connect it with the **Crown** chakra and its energy. Because the Pituitary and diencephalon are directly connected neurologically to the higher brain, the cerebrum therefore, is significant to this chakra.

This chakra is the seat of understanding.
This is where we do our true learning, –
by connecting the knowledge acquired cerebrally, (ie: the intellect) to our discernment and intuition from our instincts and the experiences of life.

The consequence of imbalance and blockage in this energy centre are:-
Sense of hopelessness; lack of ability to use foresight or judgment.

Consequently it is very important that this area is kept clear and energised to make full use of our reasoning abilities. It is our **clarity of foresight** and **ability to consider situations and people** with **awareness** that brings balance and harmony to our lives.

Do we not use the terms 'high brow' and 'low brow' to describe peoples' judgment?

WHAT

Our intuition *interprets* our instincts and thinking to enable *balanced judgment*, just as the pituitary *interprets* the hormones in the bloodstream for the body's requirements for *balanced health*.

Here we will look at the connection between this Master Gland and the cerebrum and see what negative thinking is related to the pituitary and diencephalon *function*, (both *conscious* and *subconscious*) and see how that negativity invades their energy, slowing down or blocking this centre.

When we cannot 'think straight' or work something out, do we not furrow our brow; rub our forehead? This indicates the seat of blockage and also the instinct to clear it.

The *function* of this area of the Pituitary and the Diencephalon has shown its overall control of all other endocrine glands but significantly it enables the development for the body's *changes*, the *milestones* throughout life.

There are twice the changes for women hence this energy centre, is the seat of the *feminine principle.*

- Growth to adulthood.
- Sexual maturity.
- Pregnancy.
- Cessation of fertility in women.

Emotional concepts and ideas are readily formed from the *function* of the Pituitary gland, because the pituitary deals with natural *physical* and *psychological* change. Because this is a major and complex endocrine gland, it follows that this is also emotionally complex. With the function dealing with so many aspects of reproductivity and sexuality the corresponding emotions and *associated memories* are dominated by them, especially in this modern *sexually-oriented* and *image-conscious* society

Our physical sexuality is not only naturally strongly influenced from the subconscious instinctive *urge of survival* but is a very important factor in our *sense of identity* to ourselves and other people of both sexes, regardless of sexual preferences. This is now determined both physically *and* emotionally in man because the state of the emotions has become an important factor in how we *deal* with our place and survival in society.

The emotions and thoughts involved can and do lead very easily to negative thinking.

WHY

Sources of negative energy:

Internal Physical. 1)

- Bodily changes: puberty, pregnancy, menopause.
- Hormonal **imbalances**.
- testosterone/œstrogen surges, PMT, Mood changes/swings.
- Acute and chronic 'stress' involving adrenalin.

Internal Emotional.

- Self-expectations at critical physical changes. ('growing up' 'growing old' concepts etc.)
- Distaste for periods/menstruation or sex.
- Negative memory associations.
- Sexual anxieties.
- Expected & Perceived conscious & subconcious responses from others to moods/behaviour/image/social pre-conceptions.

Internal Physical. 2)

Associated Conditions, Illnesses, Diseases of Reproductive System.

Internal Emotional.

- Self-Evaluation, a) being ill b) illness in sexual area.
- Anxieties; fears.
- Negative associations/memories of sexuality and illness in general.
- Expected & Perceived responses conscious & subconscious from others to illness/ social pre-conceptions.

These complex and strong emotions influence, if not control, our behaviour. This area is vulnerable because it is so involved with survival and identity in both normal conditions and that of illness. Our sphere of influence is much wider in today's society due to travel and communications. We are also more open to the views of a wider world.

There is also greater encouragement to strike out on one's own and the sense of family and its structure are being dismantled. Survival and sexual success are therefore not supported by the safe family group. The individual is having to carry the greater part of this responsibility and becomes burdened by it from complex negative emotions that reduce his or her energy for the purpose.

The modern concept of living in the emotions and expressing them adds to the complexity of how we react and interact in relationships and society, especially sexually. Conscious awareness of this complexity and focusing our understanding on all the aspects is how we can help both ourselves and others.

External sources.
These influences affect us strongly as well.

External Physical.

- The physical reactions to sensory organs *Sight, Smell, Touch* etc and their memory associations.

Side-effects of hormonal imbalance

- acne/spots.
- bloating.
- period cramps.
- morning sickness/nausea.
- moods/aggression.
- hot flushes.
- menorrhagia (heavy bleeding).
- weight gain at critical periods.

External Emotional.

- Peer pressure.
- Social conditioning & pre-conceptions, old wives tales.
- Responses from others to moods/behaviour/appearance.
- Sexual partners/family/colleagues' own negative agendas, triggering negative response in us.
- Physical and emotional changes in sexual relationships. (Augmented by further *thoughts* and *emotions*)
- The media in all forms, which plays to/on our emotions.

Sadly Depression, anxiety, sexual problems and issues are high in modern society so that realising the source and specific area for the sense of hopelessness and inability to think straight that we all go through in varying degrees, is essential in helping to deal with it.

Because of the changes in attitude to patterns of gender behaviour men are being urged to '*get in touch with their feminine side*'.
This has been largely interpreted or judged in two ways.

1) That men should show or express their 'softer' emotions.
   Being easier for women, this is frequently considered as 'womanly' and women as emotional creatures. Both these perceptions are negative and imply that these emotions are automatically out of control, are difficult to deal with and best avoided.
2) Seen as men doing 'female' chores.
   This can be judged as performing the female 'rôle.' Since this can lead to a confusing or undermining situation, this becomes negative and both men and women feel displaced and unable to judge or work out the dynamics of the relationship.

The '*feminine side*' however is to do with **intuition**, **creativity** and **sensitivity** to others. Being '*in touch with*' these aspects of our humanity is to round out the capable, organising side which manages the self and life's practical and financial needs, ie: the masculine principle. Thus the two 'sides' balance each other in *each person*. The **Brow** is the seat of understanding. This 'understanding' is what enables all relationships to flourish with less conflict. This answers personal needs more fully.

Therapeutic treatment and chakra clearing techniques for the Pituitary area and brow will be helpful and advisable in all conditions a client brings. However special focus and attention to them need to be given if, accompanying any physical manifestations, feelings of hopelessness or poor judgment etc, are apparent. When this remains or deepens to a sense of hopelessness etc, there will invariably be physical signs of increasing or intense negative blockage.

PHYSICAL CONSEQUENCE

for eg:

Headaches: across eyes and at the back of the head.
Muscular tension in face with knock-on effect to neck and shoulders.
Generally feeling tired/unwell.
Bad dreams.
Any conditions or symptoms locally and from reproductive system will often linger or be recurring.

Stronger or serious deep issues from these aspects would manifest problems in those areas of the body where the heavier, deep subconscious negativity has gravitated to the lower chakras.

Headaches are invariably from *muscular* tension, except in those cases of specific disease or trauma.

Any hormonal imbalances from the Diencephalon activity will increase the chances of creating negative energy in this area; so keeping it clear and energised will improve the body's ability to adjust the balance. (*See also* **Sacral** chakra, p120)

Because the Anterior lobe of the Pituitary maintains the health of the smooth muscle in the body, blood vessels, bowel, bladder etc, will all be affected by the situations and their emotional issues we have explored above as we all know.

At some time we've all had a wildly beating heart, the 'runs' or extra trips to pass water, or feeling sick, even vomiting, being hot from embarrassment or cold with fright. This is where judgment is suspended and we can hardly think straight. Adrenalin is running high and memories are being over-stimulated. We've all experienced these in and from our relationships, from falling in love to all manner of relationship upsets.

Those in the healing professions need to be aware of the involvement of emotional energy in these areas as well as any conditions and illnesses in these areas too. These invariably linger or recur if energy from these negative emotions becomes trapped preventing that free flow of natural positive energy. We need good chakra circulation to keep our vitality high.

HOW

> Healing/releasing is needed in the **Pituitary** area as well as the site of the condition or illness to give the greatest effect. Attention focused on the **Brow** chakra can greatly enhance the treatment being given.

'Positive Distraction Thinking'.
If possible, any encouragement to positive thinking and interest (and activity too), that involves the beauty in nature that surrounds us will enhance the natural energy of this chakra and will be very restorative, eg: focusing consciously on any natural aspects for example the trees, gardens and countryside etc, the easiest source around us, is an excellent quickie distraction.
How many of us instinctively seek some form of personal outdoor green activity or gardening, visits to the coast or countryside as therapeutic aids to our workaday stresses? The denial and lack of these in certain urban surroundings is self-evident in the problems and behaviour that are rife there.

WHAT

The **Brow** chakra also serves the Limbic System, because it is so closely associated by physical proximity and its autonomous or unconscious function being involved with the emotions generated by the Pituitary area. The chakra will therefore absorb some of the initial energy stemming from its activities. Intuition is man's development from instinct, the main aspect of Limbic function. Since the Limbic System is also concerned with the balancing of behaviour, perception, judgment and foresight will be involved and is very necessary for our well-being and quality of life. Negative aspects will naturally slow down or impede the energy .

This chakra also absorbs energy from the Cerebrum from associated conscious thought and memory in all Pituitary and Limbic activity. For the cerebrum is concerned with *interpretation* which is allied to perception and judgment.

Naturally the **Brow** chakra alone cannot hold all the negative energy arising from these very complex sources; so associated negative energy will involve, cloud or block the other centres. But remember, negative energy will keep them and the organs involved connected.

Although the source of the energy is from the close links of Pituitary and Limbic and cerebral activity, it is mainly those negative *thoughts* and *ideas* that need **perception**, **discernment** and clarity of **judgment,** (without which we feel hopelessness), that will collect and block this seat of **Intuition**. A residue of any negativity will remain behind as the heavier negative energy descends because the chakras are connected.
We've seen how the lower half of the body is physically involved and also, sexual hormonal activity works directly on the lower half of the body in the ovaries and testes; so the lower chakras will readily absorb the negative energy appropriate to them.

The various intensities of Pituitary/Limbic/Cerebral negative emotional energy will **gravitate** or move to the other chakras.

Different aspects will occupy *different* chakras.

- Aspects of confusion/despair will be drawn into the **CROWN** chakra.
- Tension from unspoken distress/frustration etc will go to the **THROAT** chakra.
- Sadness/'heartbreak' and Self-pity will be drawn to the **HEART** chakra.
- Anxiety/thwarted will/negative ego will block the **SOLAR PLEXUS** chakra.
- Sexual negativity/frustration etc will descend to the **SACRAL** chakra.
- Fear/anger/hatred/sense of personal inadequacy will descend to the **ROOT** chakra.

We can see clearly how the whole body is affected and involved in the effects of negative energy. This is why we feel tired and out of sorts, emotionally drained, even exhausted without really being ill. Our energy is being depleted, quite apart from inhibiting the body's abilities to heal the illnesses and physical injuries that beset us.

If the situations are long-term or extreme or have any element of physical or mental trauma, they will be both deeply hidden and affect the individual's social and sexual awareness.

As with the pineal area, working on specific issues that could be attracted to any physical conditions will aid recovery best. However, all therapeutic help for the energy system to improve its flow will naturally help the body's healing capabilities.

Rooted as pituitary function is in **survival**, deeply-felt and long-term threats to our stability (i.e material & financial insecurity; fear of authority; feelings of inadequacy/failure/disempowerment etc) leads to Clinical Depression and the consequent increase in adrenalin from the state of anxiety that occurs will lead to serious imbalance in the chronic state.

Anatomically this area is for fitness to ensure survival.
Metaphysically this area is for understanding to enrich survival.

My Personal Notes

My Personal Notes

My Personal Notes

My Personal Notes

Chapter 4. The Thyroid & Parathyroid Glands.

The next two endocrine glands are both in the throat. This region is the larynx and contains the vocal chords (or voice box). The glandular tissue lies across and around them. The largest part is the thyroid and the four small masses of the parathyroid glands are embedded in it at the back. Both have different functions which we will look at separately. Together they form a balancing act for homeostasis through the use of energy and the healthy function of nerves, muscles and tissue.

First we will look at the glands themselves and then, to put the glands into context, take a look at the basic anatomy of the larynx and the vocal chords which they lie across because emotion affects the voice and the whole throat.

2 The Thyroid Gland.

WHAT

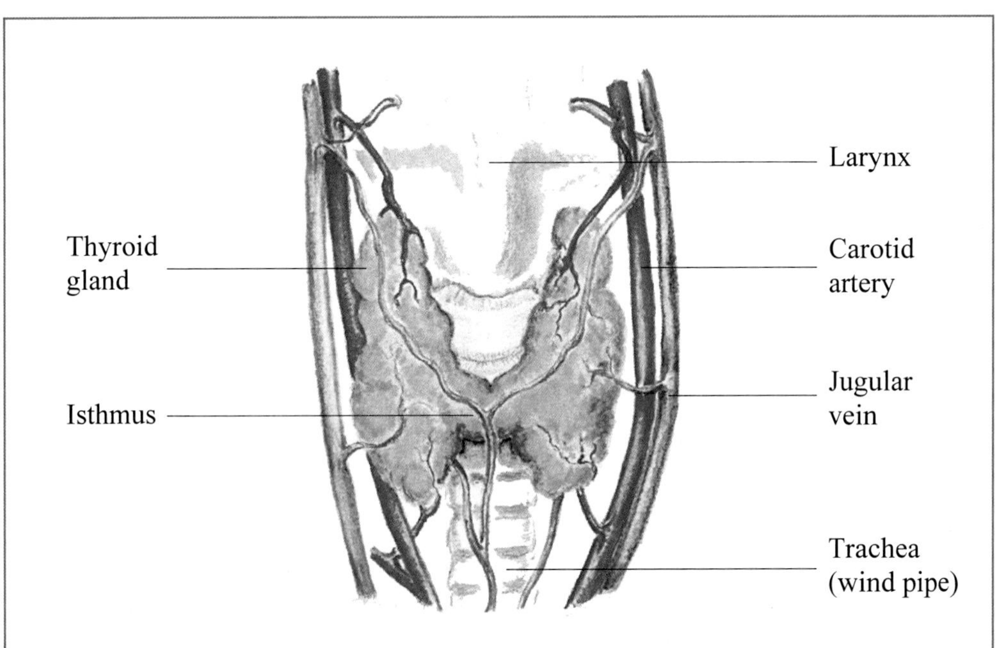

Fig:10.1. The Thyroid gland with blood supply.

This is the only gland that stores large quantities of hormones. Normally it stores about *2-3 months* supply of **Thyroid Hormone**. This shows how important it is. They are held in little follicles in a thick colloid with stored iodine which joins with the hormones. They are stored attached to thyroglobulin which is *de*tached to let the hormones diffuse into the blood when required. There they re-attach to a plasma protein for transport to target cells and are again released to diffuse into cells. They are *fat soluble,* therefore can pass through cell membrane into cytoplasm and nucleus & directly affect cell function.

The thyroid gland stores and secretes three significant hormones: the first two are known collectively as *Thyroid Hormone* as they work together.

1.Thyroxin (**T_4** with 4 molecules of iodine) is produced in greatest numbers. Acts as a spare and a back-up in the blood ready to be used.
Once **T_4** enters a cell however, it loses one iodine molecule to become the active **T_3** hormone.
2.Tri-iodothyronine (**T_3**, with 3 molecules of iodine) for fast action straight into the target cells.

Fluctuating levels in the blood act as negative feedback between the Pituitary and the thyroid gland to keep the balance correct for homeostasis.

WHY

The main function is to *regulate*:
- Oxygen use.
- Basal Metabolic Rate.

These are to do with the use of **energy.**

HOW

- Stimulates protein synthesis.
- Increases breakdown of fats.
- Enhances cholesterol excretion from gall bladder to digest fat & reduce blood cholesterol.
- Increases use of glucose for ATP.
- Maintains body temperature.
- Cellular metabolism…(cell activity).
- Growth & development (esp: of nervous tissue).

Thus thyroid hormone stimulates cholesterol in the gall bladder to digest fats into lipids which in turn carry thyroid hormone.

3. Calcitonin is the Secondary Thyroid hormone.

WHAT

This helps control the calcium content of blood ie: *de*creases blood calcium levels & conserves hard bone matrix as a negative feedback response to the action of

parathyroid hormonal activity. In this way the correct level of calcium in the blood is maintained for its various essential uses by the body: a perfect balancing act between these two glands for blood homeostasis.

The Parathyroid glands.

WHAT

They secrete **P**ara**T**hyroid-**H**ormone.

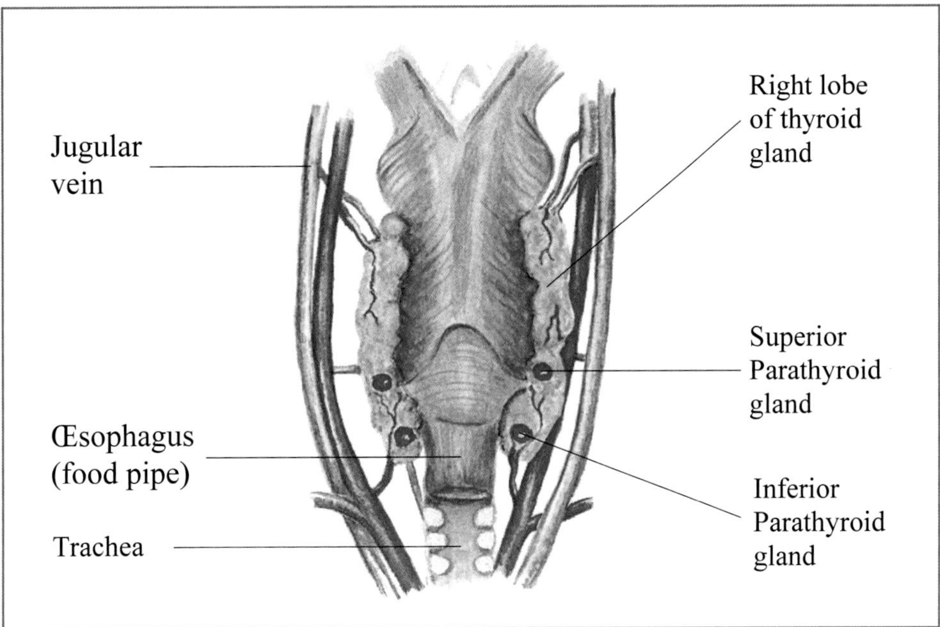

Fig:10.2. Parathyroid glands with blood supply.

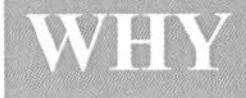

WHY

To control the release & storage of calcium levels in the blood.

Calcium in the blood is needed for:-

- Neural excitability.
- Skeletal & cardiac muscle activity and tone.
- Blood clotting.
- Cell membrane permeability.
- Proper function of certain enzymes.

Thus it is a complex and essential component covering the wide spectrum of all physical movement, strong heartbeat, accessibility to cells for nutrients and hormones, the protective device of clotting and the proper synthesis of food which all depend on it.

PTH and **calcitonin** together operate as an essential check and balance to each other by cancelling each other out as the blood calcium levels fluctuate. It is the changes in the levels that stimulate the appropriate hormonal activity to keep the correct percentage needed in the blood. This is the negative feedback operating system between **PTH & calcitonin** thyroid hormone and does not involve the pituitary.

HOW

Secretes hormone **PTH** when calcium levels are **low** and as antagonist to action of thyroid hormone calcitonin, to *in*crease calcium in blood.

- **PTH** *inhibits* bone formation and/or *dissolves old bone* (stored calcium & phosphate) to increase blood calcium when needed.
- Activates Vit D (synthesised from cholesterol molecules in the skin and stored there) for absorption of calcium into blood from food through *intestinal walls*.
- Stimulates kidneys to re-absorb calcium back into blood; the phosphates are excreted in urine.

The specialised molecules in the skin which start the synthesis of Vitamin D are stimulated by UV rays from sunlight. This stimulation occurs during daylight but is stronger in sunshine. Only as little as 15 minutes several times a week is needed, but it needs to be regular to keep up the levels. Enzymes from the liver and kidney then work on the molecules and produce *calcitriol*, the active vitamin itself. PTH then sets it to work. (People who work in artificial light for long hours and in winter especially, go to work and return home in the dark, need to be outside regularly during daylight hours.)

Because **PTH & calcitonin** hormones are secreted in response to the calcium levels in the blood, they bypass the usual stimulation from the pituitary gland.

Calcium and phosphate levels are kept regulated for *blood* homeostasis.

Now we will look at the laryngeal area and its significance to the emotional responses that affect the energy system we are exploring.

The Larynx.

This is a very muscular area with internal muscles for the structures inside and strong external muscles for the neck and head. Since the endocrine glands lie across the vocal chords, they are important to our understanding.

WHAT

1) **The Vocal chords.**

- Twin bands of vibratory muscle that cross internally from front to back of larynx just above the trachea, (windpipe). They are exercised by singers to strengthen them.

- Longer & thicker in male due to male sex hormones. This makes them vibrate more slowly, making the voice deeper. Variations in length give variety to the male voice, tenor, baritone and the deeper bass voice, both spoken and sung.

Complex intrinsic (internal) laryngeal muscles that operate the vocal chords are part of the swallowing/respiration system. Served by the *Vagus nerve.* (*See* ANS pp 138.)

Extrinsic muscles.
- The cricothyroid muscle which operates them, lies at the front of the larynx.
- Two bands of muscle fibre are attached below the 'adam's apple'.
- These divide either side of larynx to attach to floor of mouth.
- Covered in front by sternocleidomastoid muscle.
- Running from back of skull to clavicle, (collar bone).

The muscular complexities of the larynx indicate the complex muscular actions required for moving the head and throat. These actions are for obvious physical reasons and are used even more for those of *communication.*
All muscles are operated by nerves and neural responses. The nerves in the throat therefore affect the whole area as well as the vocal chords.

HOW

- The vagus nerve which has nerve endings in the throat for swallowing and the floor of the mouth for saliva production which starts the whole digestive process.
- Sympathetic nerve endings in throat counteract/shut down the vagus nerve activity when adrenalin released by emotional stimuli.
- Laryngeal muscles respond to the changes incurred in the ANS from both positive and negative emotions.
- Thus vocal chords, which are also a muscle, respond accordingly as the throat muscles tighten or relax.
- Changes to vocal tone reveals the thoughts and emotions we feel and express. If distressed or anxious/nervous/frightened, our digestive system is affected too through the sympathetic nervous system.
- ANS connects them all, *a circle of tension from throat to stomach to internal organs and back again.*

> Singers practise relaxing techniques & vocal exercises to free up the throat muscles & the vocal chords.

As we can see, the throat does not work in isolation; the connections that relate to the whole bodyare widespread thanks to the ANS and the hormone adrenalin being initiated by emotional responses.

Glossary.

ATP:…**A**denosine **Trip**hosphate…(adenine, sugars & phosphates) main energy-carrying chemical made by body to collect and store energy for use in all cells.
Basal Metabolic Rate:…rate of metabolism ie: number of calories of heat per hour (calculated at rest) that keeps the body alive and well.
Bone matrix:…calcified rigid part of bone.
Cholesterol:…lipid steroid; most abundant in body. Used to synthesise steroid hormones (eg: testosterone) and bile salts.
Clavicle:…collar bone.
Colloid:…thick fluid.
Cytoplasm:…soft gel round the nucleus of a cell containing all its necessary molecules.
Excretion:…getting rid of waste products.
Molecule:…2 or more atoms joined together.
Permeability:…having the ability to let substances pass through.
Skeletal:…to do with the skeleton/bones.
Synthesise:…to put molecules together to form a substance.
UV:…Ultra-Violet.
Vagus nerve:…large many-branched nerve supplying the digestive system. (*See* **ANS)**
Vibratory:…having the ability to vibrate and give off sound waves.

******

Associated Energy Centre for The Thyroid Gland.

Having investigated the anatomy of the Thyroid & Parathyroid glands and the larynx, we need to look at the energy associated with it and see what negative energy could come from their function that could cause problems.

Because the Thyroid gland with its parathyroid nodes crosses and enfolds the vocal chords, naturally this will be the focal point of this centre.

5th The Throat Chakra.
Seat of *communication.*
Vocal expression.
Physical expression with arms and hands.

Positive energy sources.

- **Physical**:........Normal balanced function of the gland.
  Confident vocal skills.
  Positive cerebral activity and responses.
- **Metaphysical**: **The Higher Self/Thought/Spirituality/Intuition/perception/ lovingness.**

Our ability for sophisticated verbal expression of complex thoughts and emotions is a major human factor. Through its development the vocal chords have become highly sensitive.

Not only is vocalising very important to us, playing a huge part in our lives, but we have become dependent on it. Because we rely on it so much, speech is a vulnerable skill. Discovering the sources of negative energy from the functions of the laryngeal anatomy will reveal why this area is so sensitive and vulnerable.

WHAT

The consequence of imbalance and blockage in this energy centre are:
Poor communication skills,
suppression of need and wish to express oneself freely.

When we are distressed or hurt, we are often 'stuck for words'. Or 'say the wrong thing' and make things worse.

It is emotion that stimulates communication. Emotion therefore influences the vocal chords, so it will be helpful to discover why and how this affects this area and its centre. We can then see why the throat needs healing and attention for ensuring a flow of positive energy. Both positive physical and metaphysical energy sources will make full use of our expressive abilities for our greatest benefit.

The key anatomical words for this area are.

- **Metabolism**.........ie: the use of energy.
- **Chemical balance** for nervous, skeletal and muscular systems etc.

The sophistication of all aspects of communication is matched by the complex effects of the endocrine activity of the thyroid and parathyroid, and the anatomy of the larynx. What happens in this area covers a broad spectrum physically. The throat therefore is effectively a specialised centre for the whole body.

As a consequence, the sources of negative energy come into different categories that would be helpful to explore. This will also give a clearer idea of the expressive communication needs of man and why there are physical and psychological problems that affect them and influence our lives. Understanding them is the first step to sorting them out.

Variety of aspects we will look at:-

- The use of energy.
- The vocal chords.
- The skeletal, nervous and muscular systems.
- Fat metabolism/digestive system.
- The laryngeal nerve supply connection with the digestive system.
- Adrenalin connection.
- The skin, from **PTH** activation of Vitamin D.

The whole business of communication is quite an energy-burning process involving muscular and skeletal as well as cerebral activity. Just the physical daily and constant activity in the throat involves several aspects. This increases under emotion/stress.

- *Swallowing*; constant reflex/start of the digestive/metabolic process. Under emotion/stress either difficult or convulsive (air swallowing).
- *Speech*; talking, laughing, shouting out, humming and singing etc Under emotion/stress, strained/harsh/shrill etc.
- *Neck movements*; in conversation/physical expression of communication etc Under emotion/stress, throat muscles constrict/floor of mouth tightens.

Aggressive use of the voice uses a lot of energy; stimulates secretion of adrenalin; temp and pulse increases, blood pressure rises, increased physical movements.

Negative emotions are very readily and quickly revealed through the vocal chords, so we will look first at the various sources of negative energy particularly related to the thyroid. The basal metabolic rate of each individual determined by the thyroid hormones deals with all day-to-day needs, but under emotion the metabolic rate is adapted through the stimulation of Adrenalin. This increases thyroid activity. Adrenalin (norepinephrin) is activated by emotion, and the stronger that is, the more energy is needed and burned. (*See* Chapters 8 & 9.)

HOW

Sources of negative energy. 1)

1) Internal Physical.

- Poor vocal control.
- Defensive speech which increases negativity.
- Trauma/illness to throat/vocal chords/thyroid gland.
- Poor eating habits upsetting Basal Metabolic Rate.
- *Over-activity* of Sympathetic system and Thyroid due to acute and chronic 'stress' from personal anxieties/trauma.

- Unable to speak out/defend oneself/poor ability/lack of vocabulary.
- Anxiety/Fear of speaking out - expected or perceived result.
- Sense of 'It won't change anything if I do speak out/up'.
- Sense of isolation.
- Self-consciousness/fear of humiliation.
- Expected & Perceived conscious & subconscious responses from others.
- Frustration at lack of expressive powers/opportunities.
- Negative memory associations, especially from deep past.

The voice plays an active and passive rôle in communication, depending on need and emotional mood. Energy levels play their part also.

Because parathyroid hormone activates Vitamin D stored in the skin for its calcium control, the skin's surface can manifest conditions from being unable to voice, or being prevented from voicing, emotions such as anger or frustration, self-criticism or fear. This can be either from one's own inhibitions, fear of others or humiliation of some kind. Just as vitamin D is stored in the skin, so strong emotions from this source are 'stored' in the skin.

How often are we just 'itching' to say something? Our skin even goes hot when we can't speak out or are lost for words!

The whole body itself is relevant because of the Thyroid and Parathyroid function for balancing appropriate calcium blood levels for nervous, skeletal and muscular health.

WHY

Body performance & energy levels:-

- Makes/keeps us independent.
- Determines ability to compete for 'Partner'/friends/sporting/leisure activities.
- Appearance; conforming to society's demands & conditioning.

Being in good shape, frequent physical activity and healthy eating are very strong pressures these days.

- A lifestyle for a better quality of life.
- A means to attract partners and like-minded people.
- 'Not looking one's age' for people past middle age; being trim and fit have become important strategies to hold back 'old age' and loss of independence.

Through these we communicate:-
- Our identity, consciously.
- Our *sense* of identity, subconsciously.

Finding one's place, being accepted by our peers and society enables us to verbalize freely and express ourselves comfortably; 'fitting-in' is both desirable and a pressure. Also we have the modern concept of 'being an individual' which conflicts with man's herd instinct and wish/need to conform.

Sources of negative energy. 2)

2) Internal Physical.

- Digestive system......Gastric upsets/problems/slimming fads.
- Skin.....................acute & chronic problems.
- Bones..................'crumbling of the spine', osteoporosis.
- Muscles................'cramp'/tension etc.

Internal Emotional.

- **Self-Evaluation**; 'poor specimen'/being feeble/old/weak/ill loss of identity or rôle/having 'no voice' in life's decisions.
- Guilt, Anxieties, Fears (real and perceived) on above issues.
- Slimming pressures/urges/failures.
- Expected & Perceived negative responses both conscious & subconscious from others.
- Negative associations/memories; deep past to recent/current.

As well as our internal sources, the world around us is communicating with us. Thus sources of external negativity need to be understood also.

External Physical.

- Obsessive physical training or activities.
- Not being listened to/ignored.
- Being spoken to negatively/rudely/shouted at etc.
- Hearing negative/unpleasant/aggressive verbalizing.
- Under criticism/verbal rejection/mockery etc.
- Memory associations.

External Emotional.

Partners/family/friends/associates/colleagues:-

- Affected by their own issues, *internal* associations and emotional responses causing reaction of negativity in us.
- Negative verbal outpourings from others.
- Chain-reaction from our own negativity.
- Frustration/anger at poor communication.
- Being/feeling misunderstood.
- Real and perceived criticism/verbal hurts.
- Expected & perceived view of appearance/fitness.

Overweight/obesity & anorexia where the metabolic rate is out of sync are all the physical expression of negative self-concept. The distribution of the weight indicates the areas that are the seat of the unexpressed issues. In the case of anorexia, to the individual, their whole person is 'at fault'.
The metabolic rate and adrenalin being closely interlinked, the thyroid is invariably involved in ME where fatigue and high adrenalin rushes (from sensory overload) occur, as in Clinical Depression, (*See* note p53). Communication is difficult from both physical and emotional causes so although both are linked to '*disempowerment*,' (*See* **Root** chakra p 140) issues associated with the **Throat** chakra are very relevant too.

Imagine how much spoken and unspoken negativity is 'received' by overweight/obese or anorexic people either from criticism or pity every time they are seen by anyone? How much does this increase their own negative self-evaluation?

WHAT

Just as the Thyroid gland is a *physical control* centre for the use of our energy,
the **Throat** chakra is the *metaphysical control* centre for our energy.

Proper command of the voice and good condition of a healthy body give us **control** over our lives, experiences and situations. Keeping the throat area free from negativity gives us that control.
Through positive energy we are in control of it and our lives.

WHY

Lack of control.
Misunderstandings, being misunderstood and 'not being listened to' are the cause of much distress, problems and wastage of energy.

Children, pre-pubescence and puberty.

Learning to express the new and complex, even difficult thoughts, feelings and emotions during childhood and growing-up frequently leads to young people being particularly susceptible to throat infections. Parents are often advised that 'they'll grow out of it'. They usually do as and when their communication skills develop and their hormones settle to adult levels.

HOW

Having the ability and the opportunity for expression is essential to developing positive communication skills. We need to explain and reveal what we feel and think clearly.

The proper use of *language* and *speech* is therefore essential for clear and expressive communication.

Through the use of language and communication skills we grow into our relationships and cope with the world about us. Thus we can achieve personal growth, development and make the best use of our energy. Plus, enrich our lives as a result.

WHAT

As the nerve impulses flood along the nerves, so does the emotional energy as well, stimulating the thyroid to activity for the fluctuating energy needs. Negative energy however, being heavy, gets trapped in the energy centre ie: the **Throat** chakra. When the energy here is not flowing freely, general effects are soon felt.

PHYSICAL CONSEQUENCES

for eg:

- Prone to sore throats/loss of voice.
- General tiredness/feeling off balance.
- Feeling weak/lethargic/out of shape etc.
- 'Upset stomach'/poor digestion/ poor/bad eating habits.

local conditions or illnesses (will often linger or be recurring).

Stronger or serious deep issues from all these sources, would manifest problems especially in the digestive system, (eg: irritable bowel/colitis) also metabolic issues like obesity, or chronic or re-current skin conditions.

Local problems, conditions, illnesses and diseases are not only able to develop, but the healing resources of the body are impaired. We really need to ask ourselves what are we not expressing/saying that we feel we need to, to help our body use those resources better.

If the situations are long-term or extreme, have any element of physical or mental trauma (especially where constant criticism or prevention of a person's expression has occurred), they will be both deeply hidden and affect the individual's abilities to communicate and form relationships.

HOW

Any physical manifestations in other areas of the body that are *accompanied* by any indications of communication issues and/or gastric/weight/skin problems would therefore indicate that: -

Healing is needed in the **Thyroid** area as well as the site of the condition or illness to give the greatest effect. Attention focused on the **Throat** chakra can greatly enhance the treatment being given.

Clear thinking and intuition enhance communication so attention to the **Crown** and **Brow** chakra areas will be very helpful.

All positive thinking is good, but some people can't find or accept a positive aspect to the problems they have. Even to raise them, or wish to reveal them is difficult. If possible consider/suggest that as negative thoughts come up use/try:-

'Positive Distraction Thinking.'
Thinking of or doing something pleasurable or interesting quickly instead to boost the positive energy we need to help our health and well-being.

'Positive Distraction strategies'.
An excellent quickie release and distraction strategy is focusing quickly on a favourite song, perhaps putting on a CD or finding music to sing and dance to. How often a song expresses just what we feel or cheers us up! A good burst of expressive dancing is very releasing too!

Instinctively, we can't wait to tell someone when our emotions are running high; this is our instant release valve.

Because improving communication is so essential, these might be helpful suggestions

- Consciously moderating the voice and even lowering the pitch reduces negativity in oneself and in the response from others.
- Any positive thinking plus interest (and activity too), that involves the expressive arts like singing, dancing, fun runs, yoga, Tai Chi, for example, will enhance the natural energy of this chakra and will be very restorative.

Strategies for dealing effectively with emotional ties and pain are explored in ***Section 3.***

WHY

The chakra circulation can become seriously blocked because the throat is a small area and also emotionally sensitive. However, not all the complex negative energy produced from its functions can be held in the energy centre.

> The various intensities of Thyroid/Parathyroid negative emotional energy will **gravitate** or move to the other chakras.
>
> *Different* aspects will occupy *different* centres.

- Aspects of confusion/despair will be drawn into the **CROWN** chakra.
- Hopelessness/inability to see ahead will block the **BROW** chakra.
- Sadness/'heartbreak' and Self-pity will descend to the **HEART** chakra.
- Anxiety/thwarted will, negative ego will descend to the **SOLAR PLEXUS** chakra.
- Sexual negativity/frustration will descend to the **SACRAL** chakra.
- Fear/anger/hatred/sense of personal inadequacy will descend to the **ROOT** chakra.

We can see clearly how *the whole body is involved in our communication*, as it expresses what we feel in many ways. The effects of negative energy involves all aspects and makes us feel tired and out of sorts, emotionally drained, even exhausted without really being ill. Expressing ourselves and communication is then not at its best. Our energy is being depleted unnecessarily, quite apart from inhibiting the body's abilities to heal the illnesses and physical injuries that beset us.

The Thyroid gland, although quite close to the body's surface, is protected by a highly complex set of strong muscles. This ensures a flexible area so that the energy processes of the thyroid are therefore able to work freely and aid flexibility of speech. It is this very flexibility and effortless use of this vital communication skill that gives us confidence in our relationships with people and the world about us.

Keeping this area flexible is essential, so that any work on the energy system or releasing methods to restore the circulation and flow will help to ensure this. Naturally this will help any physical or psychological healing process in this vulnerable but vital area. Being 'stiff-necked' with pride means someone is not expressing what they think or feel!

Professionals in the Expressive Arts have to be mentally & physically controlled and focused to use their energy properly, and be positive in mind to enhance their talent. We seek them constantly as an outlet to expressing life's complexities. We are happy to be spectators to their skilled use of voice and body to 'tell' us things, stir our emotions and help us recognize things about life and ourselves. We admire their focus, control and the application that have trained their skills......yet we do not usually think about focusing *our*selves and using positive energy to help us express *our*selves!

Anatomically this is the power-house of Energy.
All communication depends on some form of energy.
Metaphysically this is the power-house of communication.

My Personal Notes

My Personal Notes

Chapter 5. The Thymus Gland.

Moving down the midline of the body from the throat we come to the chest cavity. Here the thymus gland lies between the lungs at the base of trachea but at the top of the heart and protected by the sternum (breastbone).

Two-fold function.
- An endocrine gland producing hormones.
- A lymphatic gland to fight infection.

The Thymus also plays an important part in the development of the child so this is a fascinating gland that deserves understanding.

Two Stages.
The thymus produces 2 main and 2 secondary hormones. These give it two distinct stages to its life: childhood, and a gradually lessening rôle as we grow older. **It is the only gland that is very large at birth and atrophies (shrinks) to a small gland in adult life**. It is still not fully understood but this gland is very worthy of our attention.

WHAT

Pyramid shaped, Bi-lobed,
Surrounded by lymph nodes,
A protective capsule of connective tissue surrounds each lobe with an outer capsule surrounding both.

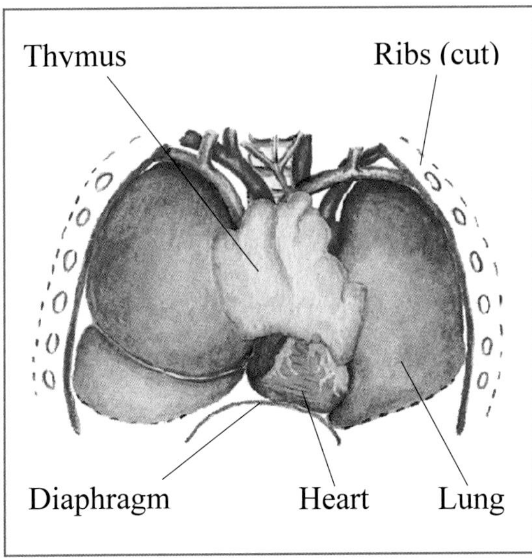

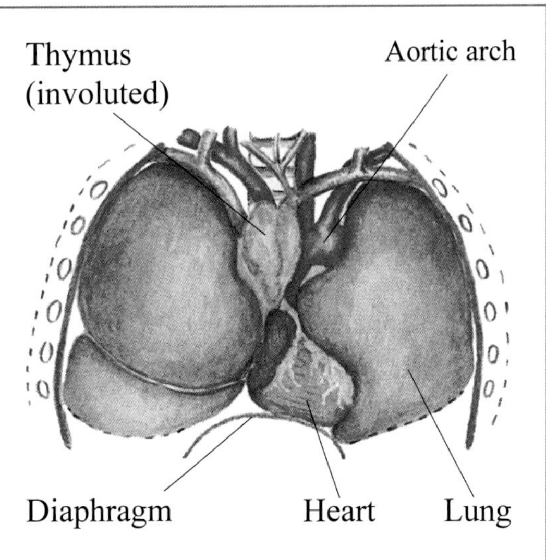

Fig:11.1. Thymus gland in **child**. **Fig:11.2. Thymus** gland in **adult**.
Large network of blood capillaries bring immature white cells (lymphoctes) via blood stream from bone marrow for development into **T cells** in the Thymus gland.

These mature white killer T cells diffuse into the large network of lymph vessels that issue from the connective tissue between the lobules of the thymus for use in and by the lymphatic system. These developed lymphocytes deal with bacteria and viruses and the toxins they produce once active in the body.

Structure.

Delicate tissue of very fine **lobules.**
Each has 2 layers:-

- **Cortex** outer layer; densely packed with lymphocytes.
- **Medulla** finer inner layer probably where hormones are produced; this develops **T cells.**

2 types.

- **cytotoxic** cells; killer cells which target specific antigens
  eg: *leukocytes* & *phagocytes* with matching receptors;
  these cruise in the blood stream, surround and digest invaders.
- **Helper T cells**; control strength and quality of all *immune responses*
  eg: *Antibodies*, which attack & digest bacteria and foreign proteins.
  Interferon, which inhibits viral reproduction.

Thus this gland plays a constant inter-active role with another system, the lymphatic system by supplying and regulating it.

Survival is the definitive function of this busy little organ, which it performs with this hugely efficient system of protection.

However, in early life when the body is most vulnerable and needy, this survival factor includes aspects of the reproductive system.
The Thymus ensures that the body is *fit for the task,*
and for its continuing survival to raise and nourish offspring.

WHY

Three known Functions.

- Development of T cells for immune system;
  stimulates *development*, *secretion* and *distribution* of T cells.
- Holds back puberty changes till body physically mature.
  Allows time for child to develop/learn sufficiently for reproductivity.
- Helps control calcium levels in blood.
  This helps control muscle tone to ensure physical equilibrium.

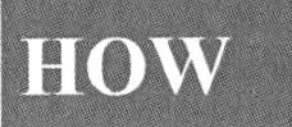

Produces two main hormones.

Thymosin and **Thymopoetin.**

- Stimulate immature white cells in bone marrow.
- Transports them to Thymus for maturing/distribution.

Thymosin is also a counterbalance to calcitonin in thyroid for calcium levels for muscle tone.
Acts as balance for chemical components for muscle tone, ie: ensures equilibrium, which in turn 'balances' body itself.

Secondary hormones.

- Thymic Humoral Factor. (**THF**)
- Thymic Factor. (**TF**)

Produced to work together as an '*inhibitor*' to the testosterone and œstrogen production needed for secondary sexual development, to allow time for the body to grow both physically and mentally mature enough for reproduction.

The two stages of the thymus are quite distinct.

From birth to puberty.
Adulthood to full maturity.

WHY

First Stage.
At birth the gland is very large.

High T cell production needed through Babyhood/Childhood.

- To counter constant invasion of bacteria and viruses.
- To stimulate antibody production virtually from scratch.

High hormone production of testosterone inhibitor.

- Needed to delay sexual maturity till body is physically mature.

As body matures:-
Antibodies stored in the blood increase over the years. Once the reproductive organs within the maturing body are developed sufficiently, production of the 'inhibitor hormone' is *stopped* so that the secondary sexual characteristics can develop by triggering *gonadotrophin* production in the pituitary.

This also allows essential time for the individual's experience of life to give enough mental and emotional development and maturity to deal with having and raising children.

By adulthood sufficient antibodies are now in supply. As the need for high production of white cells diminishes, so does the glandular tissue.

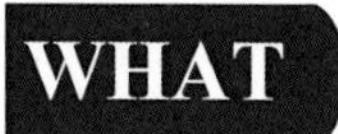

Stage two.

Once puberty is reached it 'involutes' to small gland for adult needs.

For maturing T cells & controlling blood calcium levels.

Only a small amount of tissue is now needed to sustain the immune system and help with muscle tone.

Lobular tissue is replaced by fatty tissue.
In late age most of the gland is reduced to fatty connective tissue.
This is why we become physically less toned and sometimes less able or take longer to fight infections in 'old age'.

Glossary.

Antibody:...destroys or de-activates bacterial invaders.
Antigen:...any foreign substance that activates immune system.
Bi-lobed:...(**bi-** = two)...having two lobes.
Capsule:...sac containing fluid.
Components:...contents making up an item.
Connective tissue:...binds and supports.
Equilibrium:...even balance.
Inteferon:...protein that inhibits virus reproduction.
Involute/involution:....becoming smaller by turning inward.
Leukocytes:...white cells..collective name for five types with various functions, including lymphocytes.
Lobules:...small lobes.
Lymph:...specialised fluid between cells that absorbs excess fluid and proteins and returns them to blood stream via the lymphatic vessels.
Lymphocytes:...2 types. **T**; attack infected/cancerous cells & **B**; produce antibodies.
T cells:...white cells matured in the Thymus.

******

Associated Energy Centre for The Thymus Gland.

The Thymus during childhood till puberty lies on top of the heart encompassing the upper chambers. Although involuted (reduced) in adult life it is still close to the heart. Naturally its associated energy centre is the **Heart chakra**. Through its 2-stage functions we will discover the reasons why.

4th The Heart Chakra.

Central chakra containing *passive* and *active* energy;
Seat of Love….2 elements:-

Passive…compassion.
Unconditional lovingness.
Encompassing/Generosity of spirit.
Emotional nourishment.
(giving/receiving/responding)

Active…love: affection/caring/giving of self
activates ***physical*** expressions of love.

Positive energy sources that energize this centre:-

- **Physical**:……..Normal balanced function of gland.
  Positive physical/loving activity and cerebral responses as above.
- **Metaphysical**: **Higher self**, **intuition/perception**, **being loving/lovingness** within.

WHY

Thanks to the thymus having an *inhibitor* to secondary sexual development during childhood until puberty, the individual has the time needed to gradually learn to relate and inter-relate with others while gaining the necessary communication skills and emotional control before biological sexual pressures begin.

Because Childhood is the time most dependent on relationships, this is the best time to establish these abilities to stand us in good stead as independent adults once we've left the 'security' of home, and for ensuring secure personal relationships for our own children.

The Thymus ensures this by ensuring childhood.

Only through the give and take of relationships do 'loving' and 'lovingness' grow and develop fully. This is essential to our complex relationships which indicates the significance of this gland being in the **heart** chakra. Also through inter-relating socially, the gradual perception of other's needs and feelings comes through the Higher Self to trigger compassion, generosity of spirit and lovingness to develop the inner self. The individual's value system is established in this way and determines the quality of life.

The key words for the Thymus are:-
- Protection.
- Personal development.
- Equilibrium.

Survival of the individual is still the body's biological urge. Sexuality and reproductivity being so basic to that survival, they naturally have a powerful influence. These are totally physical and remain so unless

enriched by loving/affectionate relationships through the emotions from active and/or passive lovingness.

HOW

Man has developed mentally and emotionally through living in advanced societies over millennia, therefore social aspects are as important to survival as physical ones.
- The thymus keeps us healthy and well through the auto-immune system
- The enriching aspects of our social living keeps us healthy and well through our close and loving relationships.

- *The Thymus* protects us physically.
- *Relationships* protect us emotionally and mentally.

Our *equilibrium* depends on both physical and mental/emotional health.

Having looked at the functions of the thymus, we will look at emotional concepts and ideas formed from the them and see what related negative thinking and memories both *conscious* and *subconscious*, can enter this gland's energy and invade and block this centre's circulation.

The consequence of imbalance and blockage in this energy centre are:-
Suppression/denial of affection/love/being loving.
Inability to show/feel affection/love/be loving.
Feeling afraid/unworthy of being loved.

All these aspects affect us at some stage in our lives. Any one of them complicates our relationships and this in turn complicates our lives and gives us problems and issues that cause distress and emotional pain to ourselves and those involved. When we feel any of this we can and do experience pain in the heart region. This is the contracting of this energy centre that we feel from the sudden build-up of negative energy.

The heart feels 'heavy' when we are distressed or sad, the heart is 'weighed down' by sorrow; these are always from some 'relationship' source or another!

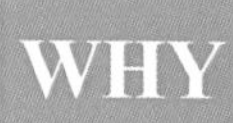

Sources of negative energy. 1)

Internal Physical.

- Poor health from auto-immune related conditions, especially in childhood.
- Poor physical tone etc.

Internal Emotional.

- **Self evaluation**;. Being ill; dependent; feeling 'different' feeling physically inadequate; rôle in family/lonely.
- Perceptions acquired Pre-puberty and Post-puberty.

Self. Negative perceptions/feelings from,

- Gender relationships, eg: parents, siblings, peers etc.
- Appearance/image in relationships/personal adequacy. (Real and Perceived)
- Social dealings/interchange/promiscuity.
- Experiences/memories/associations both conscious & sub-conscious.

Sources of negative energy. 2)

External Physical.

Health and gender related:-

- Social conditioning/demands/pressures.
- School/work environment.
- TV, media products/advertising etc.

External Emotional.

Family/Sexual partners/friends/associates/colleagues.

- Personal loss/ending of relationship(s).
- Received/perceived gender concepts in relationships.
- Family/friends/work/colleagues own *internal* relationship negativity.
- Negative responses from others to relationship behaviour/circumstances.
- Adverse pre-judgments of physical/personal value (self/others) ie: instinctive definition of 'poor specimen' syndrome' eg: late physical development, being small/'feeble'/not sporty/tough etc.
- Expected & Perceived negative conscious & subconscious judgments/responses from others.

All these negative sources will:-

- Shape our inter-relating ability and experiences,
- Determine the quality of our affectionate and loving behaviour,
- Influence our perceptions of ourselves and others in relationships,
- Affect our expectations of love and affection within ourselves and from others.

This will apply to close personal relationships and social behaviour/interaction in work and leisure situations as well, undermining our relationships and our ability to maintain and sustain relationships or make the best of situations involving others.

PHYSICAL CONSEQUENCE

- Prone to Infections/allergies.
- Lack of motivation…..general feeling of inertia/heaviness.
- Auto-immune conditions & *local* conditions or illnesses.

(will often linger or be recurring)

Stronger or serious deep issues from these aspects would manifest problems in the organs in this area as well as in those areas of the body to where the heavier deep subconscious negativity has gravitated to the other chakras. They will be kept connected through negative energy.

HOW

Any physical manifestations that are *accompanied* by relationship issues, feeling unloved, unlovable, personally inadequate, disappointed, lonely indicates that :-

Healing/releasing is needed in the Thymus area as well as the site of the condition or illness to give the greatest effect. Similar attention focused on the Heart chakra can greatly enhance the treatment being given.

All positive thinking is good, but some people can't find or accept a positive aspect to the problems they have. Even to raise them, or wish to reveal them is difficult, if possible consider/suggest that as negative thoughts come up use/try:-

'**Positive Distraction Thinking**'.

Thinking of or doing something pleasurable or interesting quickly instead to boost the positive energy we need to help our health and well-being.

Focusing on anything to do with the softer emotions, eg: kindness, lovingness around one can 'lift' the heart. Even giving oneself a pamper session will enliven this chakra as caring for one self as a conscious act for *self-value* is as important as giving or receiving affection and love from others. Giving to oneself through complementary therapies is a good way of receiving caring attention too!

Strategies for dealing effectively with emotional ties and pain are explored in ***Section 3.***

Understanding the reasons for low energy and physical problems helps us to deal with them. Not knowing increases negativity. The most important thing is to *lighten the heart*. Releasing techniques and therapeutic work on the energy system will restore the flow and ensure healthy and balanced hormonal and chakra circulation essential to this area so significant to our health and emotional life.

WHAT

The **HEART** chakra cannot absorb all the negativity that can be created from this region. Although the source of the energy is from the Thymus, it is mainly sorrow 'heartbreak', grief and negative ***thoughts, memories*** and ***ideas*** from health, relationships, self-pity and self-concepts that will collect and block this seat of **loving** and **caring.** The **heavier** energy will descend leaving a residue of negativity behind.

> The various intensities of Thymus negative emotional energy will be absorbed by the other chakras.
>
> *Different* aspects will occupy *different* chakras.

Just as the anatomical structures are inter-related and therefore connected, so are the chakras. Thus other areas of the body are affected *from* the initial source.

- Aspects of confusion/despair will be drawn into the **CROWN** chakra.
- Hopelessness/inability to see ahead will block the **BROW** chakra.
- Tension from unspoken distress/frustration will stay in the **THROAT** chakra.
- Anxiety/thwarted will/negative ego will descend to the **SOLAR PLEXUS** chakra.
- Sexual negativity will descend to the **SACRAL** chakra.
- Fear/anger/hatred etc. will descend to the **ROOT** chakra.

We can see clearly how the whole body is affected and involved in the effects of our negative emotions. This is why we feel tired and out of sorts, emotionally drained, even exhausted without really being ill, especially when a relationship ends. Our energy is being depleted so that we don't move on, quite apart from inhibiting the body's abilities to heal the illnesses and physical injuries that make us miserable or unhappy.

Relationships are the most complex of our experiences; so many emotional aspects will be involved in issues and problems that occur. If the situations are long-term or extreme or have any element of physical or mental trauma they will be both deeply hidden and affect the individual's ability to form or keep relationships or even seek them, or they become susceptible to damaging/destructive ones.

> **Anatomically** the Thymus allows for physical development and preserves our health.
> **Metaphysically** the Thymus allows for inner development and preserves our relationships.

Post Scriptum.

This observation I feel is important.

Modern society, particularly in the West has virtually abolished the rites of passage from childhood to adulthood and blurred the image of children and very young teenagers by presenting them, visually especially, as smaller versions of adults and frequently highly sexual at that. Moreover, invariably as either provoking sexuality or promising sexual activity. It also has them pursuing adult emotions and behaviour, thanks to target marketing and the media. The concept of the time-span for Childhood has changed radically.

Promiscuity, ie: frequent physical sex without relationships, is increasingly part of very young teenagers' life-style and expected peer behaviour, but they have not had time to gain either the experience or emotional development to build sustaining relationships. It is more a transitory game of social/sexual inter-change. In girls, the delicate tissue of the vagina and cervix has not matured either, which readily leads to cervical erosion. Thus the superficial sexual union in promiscuity goes hand in hand with low self-value and rejection/dismissal of love and lovingness, which infuses the gland itself and blocks the circulation of positive energy of the very chakra that vitalizes the thymus.

It seems oddly co-incidental that of the diseases that are the scourge of the modern world we have, increasingly, Asthma, Allergies and AIDS: *all of the Auto-immune system*. We have seen these increase in the last 4-5 generations, ever since the so-called 'Sexual Revolution' and the constant pressure to be both sexually active and actively sexual, which is the modern yardstick for success.

My Personal Notes

My Personal Notes

Chapter 6. The Pancreas.

Moving down into the centre of the body, we find the Pancreas. This plays a major role in the energy business as it controls sugar levels in the blood.

Although not strictly an endocrine gland, pancreatic hormones are produced in specialised masses scattered throughout the pancreas called Islets of Langerhans. The hormones are then diffused directly into the blood supply around them. These masses produce four hormones but the main one is Insulin which deals with sugar, well-known through diabetes.

Blood Sugar Levels are controlled by the **endocrine** system. Through the negative feedback system from fluctuating sugar levels, the Pituitary works with the pancreas. Adrenalin also plays its part in emergencies and under emotion, so the pancreas is an integral part of the endocrine system.

As well as being needed for all combustion in cells, *Sugar is vital to brain function*, which is why in diabetes, where the blood levels are unnaturally very low, (without enough insulin) 'going into a coma' is always a danger.

When we feel tired we instinctively talk of our 'blood sugar being low'!

WHAT

- Large soft organ.
- Behind stomach tucked into curve of duodenum under R lobe of liver, tail touching spleen.
- Well supplied with blood capillaries and nerve-network.
- Œsophageal and Peristaltic action in the stomach send impulses along *gastric* and *vagus* nerves to initiate increase in pancreatic juice via nerve network.

Sited in a flexible area of the body, the pancreas is protected by the strong muscles of the diaphragm above and the abdominal cavity, and the organs around it.

The pancreas also secretes digestive pancreatic juices. The highly acidic juices of the stomach have already started breaking down the protein ready for the further work of the pancreatic juices. These are secreted via a *duct* into the intestines; so the pancreas functions as an **exocrine** gland as well as its *ductless* endocrine function.

The breakdown of food into absorbable nutrients is the beginning of the digestive system. The pancreas is part of that. Our emotions do affect the digestion and arise from this function so a brief look at the *process* is helpful. When we know the connections, we can understand our energy systems better.

The overall function of the Pancreas is...Processing energy.

This is part of the internal energy system of the body. A brief look at how the two different functions of the pancreas inter-relate with one another will be helpful to know. Especially when we explore the connection with the Sympathetic and Parasympathetic systems (*see* Chap: 9 **ANS**.) which supplies the internal organs with nerves. It is through the ANS connection that adrenalin plays its part in the use of energy processed here.

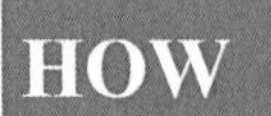

Two Functions.

1) *Exo*crine Function.
***Prepares nutrients for Endocrine function*.**

External secretion.

Produces and Secretes **Pancreatic Juice.**

- Produced in sacules of acini cells in alveolar tissue.
- Secretes digestive enzymes in high % of *water* into pancreatic ducts for discharge into duodenum.
- Secretes salt/sodium bicarbonate to make juice *alkaline*. Corrects PH of acidic chyme for enzyme action.
- One enzyme, Pancreozymin helps stimulate peristalsis. (muscular movement of walls of alimentary tract to churn and move food along)
- Part-digested fats and proteins in chyme stimulate production of Secretin from duodenal mucosa.

- **Secretin** stimulates production of *Hormone*, **Cholecystokinin.** Combines with pancreazymin for peristalsis.

Stimulates:-

- Gall bladder to release stored bile made in liver. Works with secretin to emulsify (mix with water) fat in the small intestine. This enables fat to flow through gut otherwise it would coat other food molecules and prevent their absorption.
- Flow of rich pancreatic juice.
    - Trypsin for proteins.
    - Lipase (with bile) for fats.
    - Amylase for starches. (enzyme ptyalin in saliva has started breakdown of cooked starch)

Water is essential for enzymes to break down (hydrolyse) nutrients in the chyme coming from the stomach, into simpler molecules. Amino acids (proteins & peptides) are water-soluble so can only be processed and absorbed in water.

NB insulin is water-soluble so cannot pass through the fatty membrane of cells. On arrival at its receptor, it triggers an internal enzyme (catalyst) which sets off the necessary chain of events/actions helped by G proteins. (These are on the edge or membrane of all cells and are needed to work the chemical 'switches' that makes the hormone join with its receptor to start the hormonal secretions. *See also* Type 2 Diab: p 139). With the nutrients now in an alkaline medium and split up into smaller molecules, the pancreatic hormones can get to work.

2) *Endo*crine function.

To Regulate and Balance Blood Sugar levels.

- Internal Secretion.
- Pancreatic Hormones.

Insulin, Glycogon, Somatostatin, & **Pancreatic polypeptide.**

- Produced in a myriad of scattered cell-masses (*Islets of Langerhans*); mostly near spleen.

Abundant large blood capillaries for:-

- Secretion of pancreatic hormones directly into blood stream.
- Access for *pituitary hormones* from Negative Feedback initiated by blood sugar levels to stimulate *insulin* production.

There are four specialised cell types each producing one of the hormones.

- *Alpha* cells on periphery of Islets produce **Glycogon**.
- *Beta* cells in centre of Islets produce **Insulin**.
- *Delta* cells produce **Somatostatin.**
- *PP* cells produce **Pancreatic polypeptide**.

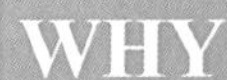

Glycogon.

***Raises** Blood Sugar Levels.*

- Stimulated by high protein intake to initiate conversion to *glucose.*
- Stimulates Liver to:-
  - Convert certain amino & lactic acids (protein & fat molecules) into *glucose.* (Liver stores it as glycogen)
  - Convert stored glycogen into glucose for release INTO blood stream.

Because the processing and use of energy is so important, it would be helpful to know that *glycogen* is also stored in muscles, the lining of the vagina & uterus for emergency use as in 'fight & flight' or very poor blood sugar levels. In extreme dieting*/starving, glycogen is not given the chance to be stored, therefore the body becomes seriously depleted of vital glucose. Also in the absence of protein in the diet, protein in muscle fibre will be converted to glycogen to supply the blood and body with glucose. This leads to loss of muscle substance. (*See* Adrenals, Chap: 8)…. *eg: anorexia

Insulin regulates Glycogon by antagonistic action thus balancing each other.

Insulin.

***Reduces** and regulates Blood Sugar Levels.*

Stimulus from:-

- Pituitary (Posterior lobe).
- Arterial glucose levels.
- Activity of vagus nerve at food intake.

Action of Insulin secretion.

- Stimulates transport of glucose, amino & fatty acids OUT of blood into tissues for combustion, especially to muscle fibres.
- Accelerates activity of enzyme glucokinase. (prepares glucose for further metabolism in cell; can be reversed for release of glucose when needed)

Antagonistic action to Glycogon:-

a) Stimulates liver to convert glucose into glycogen. *(for* storage)
b) Inhibits formation of glucose in liver from fatty and amino acids.

If insulin is not produced **B**lood **S**ugar **L**evel is too high = diabetes (Mellitus: insulin-dependent; usually starts in childhood.) Body's cells starve from lack of energy source.

- No storage of glycogen.
- No glucose into tissues for combustion.
- Too much glucose in blood; excreted into urine.
- Body burns fat instead but without glucose, combustion is incomplete = acetone in blood; excreted via kidneys and lungs. (smell of pear drops on breath) If BSL very high, causes coma, possibly death.

Somatostatin.

- Acts as *Inhibitor.*
- Regulates & balances other three.
- Stimulated by *pituitary* by blood sugar levels, inhibits the actions of the others appropriately, thus constantly maintaining correct balance.

Pancreatic polypeptide.

- Regulates the release of pancreatic digestive enzymes.
- Stimulated by high protein intake or fasting etc. (Low Blood Sugar)
- Has other unknown functions.

Because of the balancing act between the **pancreas** and the **liver**, it will be useful to look at this amazing and very busy organ and its processes to give a larger picture of the internal energy 'engine' we are exploring. Even though the liver is not part of the endocrine system, it has its connections to it and even its own hormones.

Glossary.

Chyme:…liquefied acidic stomach contents passed out to duodenum for pancreatic juices to work on.

Mucosa:…mucus membrane; lining of all cavities.

G protein:…a cell membrane protein passing signals from eg: hormones to receptor cells stimulating the interaction between them.

Combustion:...burning of oxygen & sugars to create heat & energy.

Fluctuating:…changing back & forth.

Œsophageal:…to do with the œsophagus; the food pipe.

Peristaltic:...muscular action to churn and move digestive contents along.

Catalyst:…chemical that creates a chemical change between others but remains *un*changed itself. Enzymes are catalysts.

Sacule:…little sac.

Myriad:…many.

Antagonistic:...opposite action.

******

The Liver.

This is the largest, heaviest soft organ in the body. It is a workhorse and runs like a factory with many departments. It is not an endocrine gland but because of its links to the endocrine system and internal energy, its processes are highly significant to our energy investigations.

The liver is closely connected to endocrine glands we have explored so far.

Pituitary gland:......Liver produces hormone **erythropoeitin** and is linked via negative feedback.
Thyroid gland:........Liver's metabolic processes for protein, fats and sugars. Its many activities generate a considerable amount of heat & the thyroid helps control body temperature.
Parathyroid:..........Liver stores Vit. D/cholesterol from bile for hæmoglobin.
Thymus gland:.......Specialised Kuppfer's cells in liver contain phagocytes.
The Pancreas:........Antagonistic action to control blood sugar levels.

WHAT

The liver is a ***Processing plant.*** With its vast network of specialised cells, its various activities are checks and balances to maintain homeostasis of the blood and to constantly service *the internal energy system* of the body.

- Bi-lobed, wedge shaped.
- Highly vascular.
- Protected by diaphragm above; lower ribs on right.
- Right side of stomach.
- Smaller left hand lobe partially covers stomach & gall bladder.

- Mass of hepatic **lobules.**
- No capillaries…soft-walled **sinusoids** lined with specialised cells.
- Bile channels run between hepatic cells; drain salts, pigments & bilirubin into bile ducts.
- **Bile duct** joins with **Pancreatic duct** to enter **duodenum.**

- Large **portal vein** from intestines; brings nutrients for processing.
- Large **hepatic vein** to lungs; carries away waste.
- Large **hepatic artery** from heart brings oxygen/nutrients/hormones.

Protected by the Portal sheath (loose connective tissue). This carries lymph vessels which penetrate and supply the hepatic lobules; especially Kupffer's cells which contain phagocytes to destroy microbes and render toxins harmless. These are passed into the bile for excretion and carried away in the waste from digestive system.

HOW

Activates.

- Raises blood sugar levels by:-
  - Converting stored glycogen into glucose.
  - Converting proteins & even fats into glucose if necessary.

Synthesizes.

- Oxidizes bilirubin in bile channels into *biliverdin.*
- Removes nitrogen & hydrogen NH^2 from amino acids.
  Essential to enable protein metabolism.

De-generates & Re-generates.

- Iron and globin (a protein) & bilirubin from old red cells for re-cycling.
- Dietary fats/excess cholesterol into bile salts for re-cycling for fresh hæmoglobin.
- Proteins for re-cycling from dead cell breakdown.
- Stored glycogen, vitamins & minerals for release in need.

Stores:-

- Glycogen by converting glucose.
- Vitamins A, B^{12}, D, E, K.
- Copper and iron.
- Some detoxified poisons.
- Bile in gall bladder.

WHY

Produces for export:-

- *Glucose* for raising blood sugar levels.
- Hormone **erythropoeitin** to stimulate production of red blood cells in bone marrow; in turn stimulated by *low* oxygen levels in blood if oxygen levels remain low, back-up system; kidney stimulated to produce hormone as well.
- *Heparin* to inhibit clotting of blood antagonistic (opposite; balance) to Thyroid clotting system.
- *Heat* from considerable chemical activities.
- *Bile* for emulsifying & absorption of fats in digestive system.

- *Bile salts* from fats.
- *Bile pigments* from iron & traces of copper.
- *Biliverdin* for intestinal digestive purposes.

Cleanses.

- Reduces toxic ammonia created from protein synthesis to toxic urea for excretion via kidneys.
- Detoxifies some drugs. (eg: penicillin/sulphonomides)
- Breaks down used hormones.
- Breaks down old white & red cells.

Excretes waste products.

- Urea.
- Small amount bile salts.

Thus this multi-functional organ is a whole 'organization' serving the body. The intake of alcohol and rich or greasy food will give it extra work to process it all. If this becomes a way of life or a habitual pattern then the liver will be working harder than it needs to as a constant. While it has, like the body, amazing recuperative abilities, it would be kinder to refrain from over-loading it and abusing it. Binge-drinking and late night 'Take-aways' certainly do this.

Understanding its amazing capabilities should make us respect it.

Because of the importance of energy in our understanding of the body, we will now look at the large soft organ on the other side of the pancreas, **the spleen** to complete the picture of these interactive organs. Here we can see them in relation to one another.

WHERE

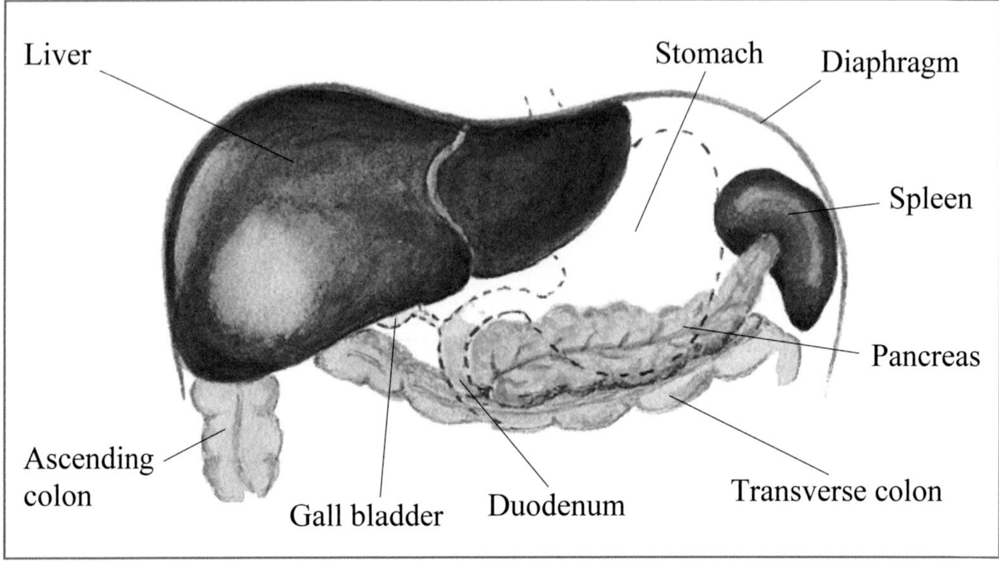

Fig:12. Relationship of the Liver, Pancreas & Spleen.

Glossary.

Bile:...mix of lecithin and bile salts.. Helps stimulate intestinal peristalsis to carry waste products away for elimination. Lack of bile lets fats coat other nutrients and prevents absorption. Protein is left undigested.
Connective Tissue:…fine tissue between. Most widespread tissue in body.
Emulsifying:…fat dissolved in water.
Lobules:…small lobes.
Oxidizes:…addition of oxygen.
Phagocytes:…engulf bacteria to digest them.
Sinusoids:…small sinuses.
Synthesizes:…forms by linking several molecules into specific groups.
Vascular:…well-supplied with blood vessels.

******

The Spleen.

It will make a helpful connection to take a brief look at the Spleen. It is not an endocrine organ, but it is stimulated by **adrenalin** and thus connected to the endocrine system, both through the Pituitary and the Sympathetic Nervous System.

The spleen deals with the blood and *maintains oxygen levels* in the body. Oxygen is vital for energy as it is used for combustion with sugar for all cellular activities. Looking at the spleen's processes for the energy system is appropriate to our theme and will show that oxygen too, is kept in balance for the body's homeostasis.

The Spleen lies opposite the liver and has similar processes for its own particular functions. Unlike the liver, the body can cope without it if it has to be removed. This shows how amazing the body's recuperative powers are in its programming to maintain homeostasis. The body will find a way if it can.

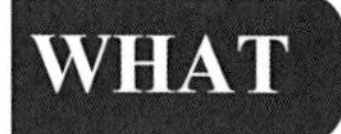

Spleen.

Associated endocrine activity:-
Stimulated by **Adrenalin,** initiated by **Pituitary** for normal activities.
Stimulated by **Adrenalin** by the **ANS**, via spinal cord short-cut, in emergencies.

2 main functions.
Processes *hæmoglobin* in blood to maintain/sustain oxygen levels.
Stores blood to restore and balance oxygen levels and blood volume.

Structure.

- Largish very soft organ on *left* side of abdomen.
- Partly under stomach.
- Protected by diaphragm above & lower ribs to left.
- *Highly vascular* lymph organ.

Splenic artery branching into widespread network.
Splenic vein branching out into many sinusoids.

***All** body's blood passes though spleen every 1½ hours.*

- In a capsule of fibrous tissue.
- Some muscle fibres.
- Regular rhythmic contractions for variations in volume to *release stored blood.*
  - Stimulated by *reduced* oxygen levels in blood.
  - Pituitary stimulates Adrenals to release adrenalin.
  - Adrenalin activates **splenic** muscle fibres to *increase* contractions to release necessary blood.

HOW

Functional tissue (parenchyma).

White pulp.

- Thick mantle of lymphoid tissue surrounds branching arteries.
- Forms uniformly scattered densely-packed nodules. (called Malpighian corpuscles)
- Blood vessels nearby.
- Contains phagocytes & leucocytes. (*See* Thymus, p75)

Red pulp.(storage)

- Held by fine supporting network of elastic fibrils.
- Intersected by fine soft-walled arterioles and vacuoles.
- Walls contain special phagocytic cells.

WHY

- Phagocytes ingest disintegrating *red corpuscles.*
- Blood seeps easily through loose-celled walls.
- Back-flow prevented by ellipsoid cells.
- Interstitial spaces filled with highly concentrated red blood cells.
- Some leucocytes.

These interstitial spaces drain into venous sinuses which have sphincters for releasing blood into **Splenic vein,** for transport via heart for eventual oxygenation in the lungs.

The Pituitary sends messages to stimulate the adrenals; adrenalin is dispatched along the nerves from the Sympathetic Nervous System (**ANS**) in neuro-transmitters to stimulate the splenic nerves. (*See* Chap: 9 the **ANS**) This initiates the reflex contractions for engorgement & dilation of spleen for continuous blood flow and any extra needed to top up oxygen levels from cellular activity.

In emergencies,

1) Hæmorrhage (Bleeding)

Sympathetic Nervous System stimulates adrenalin via spinal cord short-cut to initiate release of stored blood to replace what has been lost and keep up the oxygen levels, both to answer stress needs and correct oxygen imbalance from blood loss.

2) 'fight or flight'

Sympathetic Nervous System stimulates adrenalin via spinal cord short-cut to initiate release of more blood to provide more oxygen for all the organs involved but especially for the heart and the muscles to deal with the emergency. (*See* The Adrenals Chap: 8)

Thus strong emotions like fear and excitement engage yet another organ playing its rôle in the body's health and one moreover, dealing with the blood that *visits every cell.*

As the blood enters and flows through the spleen it undergoes several processes.

Here we will see the full range of the spleen's functions.

WHAT

De-generates; Re-generates.

- Disintegrating blood cells & platelets.
- Proteins from degenerate cells.
- Iron, copper traces, globin, bilirubin for re-cycling.

Synthesises.

- *Hæmoglobin* for fresh red corpuscles. (to carry oxygen)
- Lipid metabolism.

Produces.

- Antibodies.
- Bilirubin for bile-production in liver.
- White corpuscles from reticular stem cells in lymph.

Stores.

- Reservoir of blood for top-up or emergency.
- Lipoids, especially if high cholesterol intake.
- Iron for hæmoglobin.

Activates.

- Release of blood to increase volume/oxygen in need.

Defends.

- Destroys invaders.
- De-activates toxins.

Through a constant conditioning cycle repeated every 1½ hours, the blood is enabled to fulfil its own functions for every part of the body.

Through this cycle, whatever is happening to the rest of the body will pass through the spleen.

******

Glossary.

Arterioles:...smallest branches of arteries.
Capsule:...sac containing fluid.
Corpuscle:...literally ‘small body’.
Degenerate:...to break down.
Dilation:... widen.
Disintegrating:...breaking up.
Ellipsoid:...slightly flattened oval shape.
Engorgement:...filling up.
Fibrils:...very fine fibres.
Hæmoglobin:...protein with iron in red blood cells that carries oxygen.
Leucocytes:...white blood cells that kill viruses & some tumour cells.
Lipoid:...pertaining to fats & oils.
Neuro-transmitters:...chemical substances that pass messages from one neuron to the next.
Pathogens:...micro-organisms causing disease.
Phagocytes:...white blood cells that surrounds & digests pathogens.
Sinusoids:...small collecting place for fluids.
Sphincter:...circular muscle at a natural opening that opens at closes when stimulated to let substances in & out.
Vacuoles:...little membrane sac to hold or store substances.
Vascular:...pertaining to or having many blood vessels.

NB.... Infection inhibits formation of hæmoglobin. Formed from a pigment, **hæmatin**, comprising iron, traces copper, thyroxin, Vit C and the protein, **globin.**

******

Associated Energy Centre for The Pancreas.

Here we will look at the energy centre associated with the Pancreas. It is the **Solar Plexus** chakra. The Pancreatic function in controlling our sugar levels is central to our energy output and the solar plexus area is physically central to the torso. Solar energy, is appropriately, pure combustion.

However, the three organs we have looked at, lying centrally across the anatomical solar plexus, are all concerned with energy and combustion.

- **The pancreas....sugar.**
- **The liver.........sugar.**
- **The spleen......oxygen/iron.**

Closely inter-related as they are, they are included in the equation for this chakra.

3rd The Solar Plexus Chakra.

Seat of **Intellect, Will, Ego**.

- Masculine *principle/concepts.*
- In women this manifests in the workplace or any areas of responsibility/leadership.

Positive energy sources that energize chakra:-

- **Physical**:........Normal balanced function of the gland/organs.
  Positive cerebral activity and responses/reasoning as per above.
- **Metaphysical**: **The Higher Self/Thought/Spirituality/Intuition/Enlightenment.**

- The **liver** is the seat of **masculine energy;** it is the Processing Plant for the body's '*Provisions*'.
- The **spleen** is the seat of **feminine energy;** it deals with the *Life-giving* elements, Blood and Oxygen.

Thus the energy from both genders lies on either side of the pancreas. And this being the physical energy centre for the body, they are all involved in the energy from the strongest of the metaphysical drives in Man; the **Will**, the **Ego** and the **Intellect**.

These three elements are highly complex and inter-related, as are all the functions of these three organs. As a consequence, the sources of negative energy will come from the functions of all three organs and any negative energy build-up in them and this vigorous centre will therefore affect them all, relative to their specific functions.

WHAT

The consequence of imbalance and blockage in this energy centre are:-

Anxiety, dissatisfaction, lack of will-power/motivation.

The key anatomical words for this area are:-

- **Processing of sugar**………...control of energy.
- **Oxygen balance**……………control of combustion.
- **Breakdown of substances**….source of energy.

The functions of all three organs show this area as one of preparation, and making ready and available the body's energy sources and the nutrients ingested.
Through these processes we will look at the sources of negative energy that darken and hamper this centre so that we are either ill-prepared or even not prepared for our best efforts either mentally or physically.

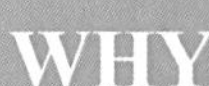

Sources of negative energy. 1)

1) Internal Physical.

- Indigestion etc.
- Comfort food binges.
- Food/alcohol overload.
- Not eating.
- Junk eating/poor dietary habits.
  - all compounded if habitual.
- Conditions, illnesses and diseases of organs involved.

Internal Emotional.

- **Self evaluation**…guilt/regret/disgust/out of control/weak-willed.
- Obsessional cravings.
- Negative reasoning/self-delusion/need for assertiveness through Will.
- Nervousness (short term) about 'performance'/ability/situation etc.
- Anxiety (long term) as per above.
- Feeling starved of comfort/attention/care, ie: neglected.
- Perceived or real inability to grasp information/task/studies etc ie: 'mental indigestion/stodginess'.
- Feeling inadequate/stupid/being in the dark/slow. (as per above)
- Negative memories and associations.

We say we can't 'digest' something when we can't or feel unable to, grasp something we are trying to learn.
When we can't stick to a task we say our 'blood sugar is low'.

Sources of negative energy. 2)

2) Internal Physical.

- Hyperventilating.
- Panic attacks.
- Extreme fatigue.
- Blood conditions/diseases.

Internal Emotional.

- Feeling 'suffocated' by situation.
- Feeling as if you are being 'bled dry'.
- Feeling 'bloodless'.
- Expected & perceived negative responses/reactions both conscious & subconscious from others.
- Negative associations/memories.

People often say 'I think I need some iron tablets or a tonic' when they feel under par.

As well as our internal sources, we are involved with other people's energy. Thus negativity that we receive from external sources needs to be understood also.

External Physical.

- Inducements for sugar comfort/junk food/alcohol. (commercial/media/social)
- Social conditioning for 'I can have what I want' etc.
- Negative information.

External Emotional.

Partners/family/friends/associates/colleagues/employer:-

- Affected by their own issues, *internal* associations and emotional responses causing reaction of negativity in us.
- Under dominant will of any of the above. (bossiness/bullying/manipulation/emotional blackmail)
- Chain-reaction from our own negativity/negative Will.
- Subconsciously inviting/expecting being under-mined/over-ruled/dominated.

All tied to negative memories and associations.

It can be seen how our **Will** and **Ego** are subject to the responses and energy of the Will and Ego of others, and our own Ego, the 'I want/must have' aspect, given attention and inducements to indulge and give in to ourselves. When either or both of these dominate, our intellect loses its influence from its reasoning powers. Our mental energy is being not being productive. (*See* **Energy is The Key,** p197)

Becoming an honest observer of any ego/will creations we have manifested for ourselves will give a clearer view to us of what we are setting up, or have set up for ourselves. These create a vibration that then interacts with others.

Is it our will and ego that initiates these or is our will and ego responding to other people's creations? If we are responding, then we have the magnet for them! Thus it is our issue too because we have attracted it to us.

This then becomes a *control* cycle. Your ego/will/desire perpetuates that situation. *Their* acceptance of it controls your ego/will creation. You each control the other.

Assessing the creations and the things they have hooked onto in us will enable us to see ourselves and others more clearly. This knowledge can really help to resolve situations and relationships that have become problems, burdens and the cause of stress and unhappiness. All of these undermine our health.

This is the highest of the three physical energy centres. The Masculine and Feminine energy it is flanked by closely inter-relates with it. These pertain to both genders.

Masculine energy that should be considered:

• Money……………..1) drive for,
2) pressure/need for,
3) lack of.

• Responsibility……...1) overload,
2) denied/taken away.

• Power……………...1) passive & aggressive dominating,
2) being dominated.

• Lust/desire…………1) material belongings, image.
2) sexual.
((both) drive/social pressure for/lack of, frustration)

Feminine energy that should be considered :

• Nourishing/caring….1) over-doing.
2) lacking,
(from others: to self)

• Creativity…………..1) Fertility: drive/primary energy channeled to have children,
2) Artistic: denied/suppressed.

• Intuition…………….1) denied/mocked/challenged,

• Wisdom…………….1) denied/mocked/challenged.

While masculine and feminine energies relate to both genders, the aspects will depend on which is relevant to or taking precedence in their personality/area or way of life.

These are all related to the Will and Ego.

Thwarted Will which is Will/Ego will enter the energy of the liver.
Because the liver is a major source of heat, fiery anger will be readily drawn to the energy here.
Power against others or the Self is Will/Intellect and will enter the physical Solar Plexus.
Nourishing and Creative issues are Will/Ego but will enter the energy of the Pancreas and Spleen.
Intuition/wisdom issues are Will/Intellect and will enter the physical solar plexus.

The denser energy from all these issues will go to the relevant chakra, **Sacral** or **Root**.

We can see how powerful the physical Solar Plexus area is from the energy of the four dynamic organs lying across it. Also, how the *three lower* energy centres are *dominated* by the Will/Ego/Intellect if these are negatively driven.

The fear of being thought stupid, 'not good enough', a failure, is very much attached to the **Solar Plexus** chakra. Poor self-concept is naturally to do with the Ego: how we see ourselves. The Will is involved because in low self-value, one is against oneself.

'Losing face' is very much a masculine fear. Because it is attached to the 'macho' idea of succeeding among one's peers, boys and young men are more likely to have this fear than girls. If a boy feels he might fail or not be good at something, it is likely that he will lose interest, pretend to have no interest or refuse to do something rather than 'show himself up', be perceived as 'stupid' or a failure. This is to act against the self.

It undermines self-confidence very seriously. We all need this to succeed and realize our potential, *especially* the young.

Being called '*stupid*' is very common. It is very frequently the first word of denigration of the young by both their peers and even parents.

This is very damaging. In the current social climate 'being successful' has created an even greater pressure, especially upon the young.

- From the media.
- From social expectation.
- From the trend of living separated from the family (supportive) group.

Being a 'celebrity' equals 'success'. This involves *money* and *image* as well. Both are to do with the Ego and the Will/I want/must have. This has added to the fear of not being adequate and turns the Ego and Will towards negativity very readily.

We need seriously to question these aspects, not only for ourselves as adults, but for the young, especially boys who are particularly vulnerable to the face-saving belief.

Through understanding the issue of '*in-case-I-look/sound-stupid*' syndrome with reference to poor behaviour or lack of progress in the young (boys especially), it is possible to realize their poor self-concept and serious lack of confidence. Once acknowledged, choosing to deal with it by using releasing techniques or even by frank discussion, if this is possible, will do much to change this damaging negative self-view.

There will naturally be connections here to the **Throat** energy centre since expressing this is invariably suppressed. This inhibits articulation too. Naturally the **Heart** energy will be involved so linking up with these other underlying issues and factors will also help to change this situation around. Since self-image/identity are also involved, issues from the **Root** area could come into the equation as well.

The anatomical and metaphysical solar plexus are centrally situated in the body. These factors are central to the demeanour we have that determines our quality of life. This is why it is so involved with other chakra energy. It does need our serious consideration because lack of self-confidence and self-value lead to seeking *dependencies*, (see pp 247/8) either from people, institutions or food/drink/drugs. (*liver*), creating subtle demands of others. Thus the intellect is used negatively. Combined with emotional energy, this becomes a very potent force that can be destructive at very subtle levels.

HOW

PHYSICAL CONSEQUENCES

for eg:,

- Prone to nervous stomach/indigestion/bloating etc.
- General tiredness/heaviness, not wanting to bother.
- Feeling drained/stodgy.
- Extra weight carried in the solar plexus area/comfort eating.
- Tension and pain across area.
- Restless/fidgety even though tired.
- Food doesn't satisfy appetite/loss of appetite.

local conditions or illnesses. (will often linger or be recurring)

Stronger or serious deep issues from all these sources could manifest problems especially in the upper digestive system or in chronic weight issues. Local problems, conditions, illnesses and diseases are not only more able to develop, but the healing resources of the body are more impaired too.

If the situations are long-term or extreme or have any element of physical or mental trauma, they will be both deeply hidden and affect the individual's abilities to control their energy appropriately. This can lead to very complex situations and even aggressive attitudes and behaviour that cause even more problems and cycles for that person.

HOW

Any physical manifestations even in other areas of the body, that are *accompanied* by any indications of anxiety, lack of will-power/motivation and you/the client feeling you/they are lacking 'nurturing,' or life is not 'satisfying' would therefore indicate that:-

Healing is needed in the **Solar Plexus** area as well as the site of the condition or illness to give the greatest effect. Attention focused on the Solar Plexus chakra can greatly enhance the treatment being given.

Clear thinking and intuition enhance reasoning, will-power and learning; so attention to the **crown** and **brow** chakra areas will be very helpful.

All positive thinking is good, but some people can't find or accept a positive aspect to the problems they have. Even to raise them, or wish to reveal them is difficult. This is especially so for people with ego and will issues. However, if possible, consider /suggest that as negative thoughts come up use/try:-

'Positive Distraction Thinking'.
Thinking of or doing something pleasurable or interesting quickly instead to boost the positive energy we need to help our health and well-being.

All positive physical and mental activities and challenges where energy is being used and focused enhances this centre. Also eating interesting, well-balanced, attractive food in pleasant, cheerful/happy surroundings/company will do wonders. (*See* p152, **ANS**)

In a society where 'stress' is endemic, 'eating out' is the no:1 leisure pastime!

Strategies for dealing effectively with emotional ties and pain are explored in ***Section 3*** with various methods to choose from to suit different situations and problems.

WHAT

With all the powerful energy produced and processed in this area the Solar Plexus chakra can become seriously blocked and easily overloaded from all the negative energy produced from the functions of the Pancreas, Liver and Spleen.

The various intensities of Pancreas, Liver & Spleen negative emotional energy will **gravitate** or move to the other chakras.

Different aspects will occupy *different* chakras.

- Aspects of confusion/despair will be drawn into the **CROWN** chakra.
- Hopelessness/inability to see ahead will block the **BROW** chakra.
- Tension from unspoken distress/frustration will block the **THROAT** chakra.
- Sadness/'heartbreak' and Self-pity will be drawn to the **HEART** chakra.
- Sexual negativity/frustration will descend to the **SACRAL** chakra.
- Fear/anger/hatred/sense of personal inadequacy will descend to the **ROOT** chakra.

This complex area with its many issues will benefit greatly from all releasing and therapeutic help for both specific conditions that will attract related emotions and the body as a whole by enhancing the energy flow to restore vitality.

Nothing runs without the appropriate fuel. Physical and metaphysical 'nourishment' for energy and survival are central to existence. Just as the body takes in food to nourish it, for energy, health and survival needs, so the mind takes in food: eg: information and knowledge for 'mental' energy, looking after the body, survival tactics and strategies.

Just as the sun beams, warms and energizes, so the energy from the Will, Ego and Intellect should beam warmly outwards to enable us to lead fulfilled, interesting lives and enjoy balanced loving relationships.

Anatomically this is the Refinery for Energy.
Metaphysically this is the Refinery for the Self.

******

My Personal Notes

My Personal Notes

My Personal Notes

Chapter 7. The Ovaries & Testes.

Moving down into the pelvic cavity, we will now look at the endocrine glands of the reproductive organs. The ovaries and testes produce hormones for **sexual development** and **function** and ova and sperm for **reproduction.**
We will look first at the ovaries as they are situated within the pelvic cavity with the rest of the female reproductive organs. The size and shape of shelled almonds, they are tucked in closely to the fallopian tubes, which lead down to either side of the uterus.

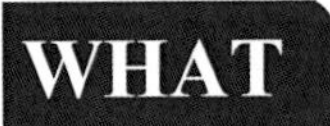

Two Ovaries.

Structure.

- Thin outer layer.
- Deep protective layer; **Tunica albuginea.**
- 2nd deep layer; **Stroma.**
  - Outer dense **cortex;** contains **ovarian follicles** with immature oocytes.

- Attached to uterus via a ligament set into the Broad Ligament.
- Attached to pelvic wall by suspensory ligament.
- Hilus, point of entry for blood vessels & nerve supply.
- Finger-like projectiles (*fimbriæ*) from the fallopian tubes hang over ovaries to receive ripe eggs, with one fimbria serving each ovary.
- Contain stem cell oogonia in follicles for development into female **gametes; ova (eggs).**

WHY

Function.

- Production of **ova** (singular = **ovum)** = Oogenesis.
- Produce **œstrogens;** female sex hormones.

Primarily **œstrodiol, œstrone & œstriol.**

- Development & cyclical functioning of female reproductive organs.
- Secondary sex characteristics.
- Fluid & electrolyte balance.
- Protein anabolism to develop oocytes into ova.
- Psychological outlook.

Secondarily **Progesterone.**
Prepares:-

- Endometrium (lining of uterus) for embedding of fertilized egg.
- Mammary glands to lactate (produce milk).

Because the ovaries have three stages of development, it is helpful to have a brief understanding of them and of how the ova (eggs) are **1)** made ready for fertilization. **2)** menstruated if not fertilized.

HOW

Ovarian changes.

- *Before birth*; primary oogonia develop in ovaries.
- *Childhood*; primary follicles develop.
- *From Puberty*; *Theca* cells develop in these follicles to produce **androgen** steroid. Stimulated by the pituitary, granulosa cells then convert androgen into **œstrogen** for development of secondary follicles ie: *Graafian follicles* and oogonia into oocytes , as menses begin. (*See also* Chap: 3 on The Pituitary & Chap: 5 on The Thymus.)

Ovulation and possible fertilization of ova.

Low levels of œstrogen and progesterone in the blood stimulates the hypothalamus to trigger the Pituitary to produce and release **FSH** and **LH** for the menstrual cycle.
FSH sets off the development of a Graafian follicle in the ovary.

LH develops it further plus triggering progesterone to stimulate the milk glands and thicken the endometrium, ie: the uterine lining to prepare for possible pregnancy

Oogenesis: stages of egg development.

1) Grows and rises to surface:-

- *Graafian follicle*;(pouch) starts rising to surface of ovary secreting **œstrogens** + small amount **progesterone** and fluid to surround developing oocyte.
- *Corpus Luteum;* mature follicle with oocyte in fluid sac (antrum); produces **progesterone, œstrogens, relaxin & *inhibin*** *which halts final stage* of ovum.

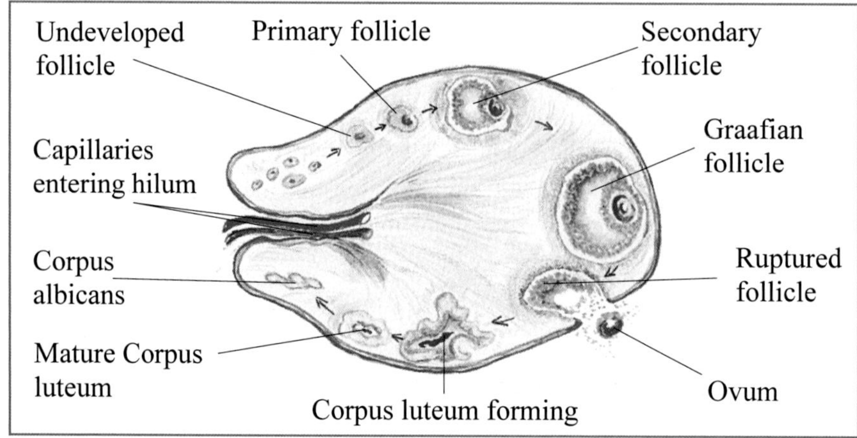

Fig :13. Stages of oogenesis.

2) Released into appropriate fallopian tube:-

- *Corpus Hæmorrhagicum;* ruptures[1] to expel ripe ovum (**ovulation**) towards fimbriæ of fallopian tube.
- Propelled along to uterus by peristalsis & moving cilia. (hair-like fibrils)
- Hormone levels drop, *inhibiting* pituitary hormone production. (**F**ollicle **S**timulating **H**ormone & **L**utenizing **H**ormone)
- Outer layer of ovum; *zona pellucida,* thick film which contains peptides to attract sperm.

3) Final stage.

1) Occurs once ovum fertilized by sperm in fallopian tube. [2]

- *zona pellucida* de-activated; fertilized ovum becomes *zygote.*
- Embedded in endometrium.
- Develops placental tissue from *zygote.*
- Secretes hormone **HCG H**uman **C**horionic **G**onadotrophin[3] .
  This stimulates *Corpus Luteum* to *continue* secreting hormones inhibited by lack of **FSH** & **LH** from pituitary at ovulation.

As placenta develops, it takes over œstrogen & progesterone production itself.
Corpus luteum then degenerates.
The developing **zygote** then stimulates Lactotrophin and prolactin in the **Pituitary** to inhibit FSH and LH to prevent oogenesis during pregnancy.

2) If fertilization does *not* occur:-

- *Corpus Luteum* degenerates into *Corpus Albicans;* fibrous remains leave tiny scar on Tunica albuginea layer.
- Endometrium & ovum expelled (menstruation).

Cycle of oogenesis then resumes as levels of FSH and LH drop sufficiently to trigger the hypothalamus and the Pituitary again.

Thus the Pituitary is in a loop of influence for both menstruation and pregnancy through production and inhibition of the appropriate hormones due to their levels in the blood.

[1] Sometimes a tiny capillary ruptures also, spurt of blood in peritoneum causes sudden severe pain = Mittleshmertz. Lasts till blood re-absorbed; approx 1-2 hours.
[2]If *Zygote* continues developing in fallopian tube this is an *ectopic pregnancy.*
[3]It is **HCG** that shows up in early pregnancy tests.

******

Now we will look at the male reproductive glands, the testes. They are supplied with seminal fluid by the prostate gland for the sperm to swim in. The prostate gland is just below the bladder and therefore in the pelvic cavity, but the testes are suspended outside the body in the scrotal sac to maintain their temperature a few degrees less than normal body temperature.

WHY

The temperature needs to be kept constant to ensure production & survival of the sperm. The ANS controls this by contraction and relaxation of the scrotum to regulate the temperature. In cold conditions the testes are reflexly drawn up close to the body or even into the body cavity to maintain the correct temperature. (Momentary fear or severe apprehension can trigger this *involuntary* inversion as a protective device. This is activated by the release of adrenalin via the ANS.)

WHAT

Testes.
Before birth they develop in the abdominal cavity and descend into the scrotum by the eighth month. Sometimes this is delayed until after birth but they need to be down well before puberty for temperature control to ensure fertility.
Adult testes.

Structure.
- Dense white fibrous capsule.
- Internal *lobules* (2-300) containing several seminiferous *tubules* each contain spermatogenic cells in various stages of development.
- Between tubules, Leydig cells produce **Testosterone.**
- Epididimus…exiting duct for sperm.

WHY

Function.
Produce *androgens* **Testosterone** & hormone **Inhibin.**
Enzyme action converts cholesterol into **testosterone,** stimulated by **LH** from Pituitary; anything between 6-12 mg per day.
Spermatogenesis:-
- Specialised cell divisions (meiosis) and crossing-over of genes mean sperms develop as individuals for vast genetic variations.
- **Meiosis** changes spermatogonia through three stages into *spermatocytes*, then *spermatids* & finally *spermatozoa* (plural).
- Become spermatozoa when head, midpiece & tail fully develop.
- Tail drops off as spermatozoon (single sperm) penetrates ovum.

The main hormone produced is **Testosterone**, the most important male hormone. It is also readily associated with sexual drive and various emotional responses. Since its functions generate considerable physical and emotional energy, it is therefore very relevant to our understanding of our energy systems and its effects. It inter-relates with the Adrenal glands, both for androgens and adrenalin.

It has three main reproductive functions in men:

1) It controls the stages of development and growth of the reproductive organs from fœtus through infancy, then puberty to adulthood.
2) The development of sperm for reproduction.
3) Maintenance of health/function of reproductive system, including growth and size of prostate gland for seminal fluid and ejaculation.

These are complex stages and effects but we will have a brief look at them as testosterone plays a dominant rôle in human relationships and society.

Testosterone.

Functions.

- *Primary* sexual characteristics ie: reproductive system/genitalia.
- Plus aiding secondary sexual characteristics.
- Protein anabolism to develop spermatagonia into spermatazoa.
- Controls condition/function of male reproductive system/personality.

1. *Before birth*; development of male reproductive system and organs.

- Some androgens are converted to œstrogens for development of certain regions of the brain.

2; *From Puberty*; inhibiting hormone from Thymus ceases.
Gonaotrophin thus stimulated in pituitary.
Testosterone increases & with **DHT*,** develops/enlarges sex organs;
Initiates:-

- Spermogenesis.
- Libido & sexual behaviour.
- Psychological outlook.
- Secondary sexual characteristics.

- Muscular/skeletal growth:
ie: wide shoulders, narrow pelvis; *androgens* are anabolic; stimulate protein synthesis which increases bone mass & heavier muscle in male.
- Body/facial hair.
- Increased sebaceous glands.
- Thickening of skin.
- Enlargement of larynx; vocal cords lengthen; subsequent voice changes.

Once adulthood is reached the main activity is for reproduction and the maintenance and homeostasis of the testes and prostate gland.

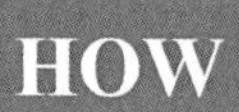

Spermogenesis.

Tubules.
- Outer layer**;** Tunica albuginea.
- Inner layer; seminiferous epithelium.

1. Immature **Spermatogonia cells** develop into male gametes; **sperm.**

2. Clusters of *interstitial* **Sustentacular (Sertoli) cells** between:
- Produce *androgens* **Testosterone** & hormone **Inhibin** (regulate sperm production via stop/go on **Pituitary hormones**).
- Produce fluid for sperm transport and to carry hormones.
- Protect, nourish developing sperms.
- Destroy excess cytoplasm.
- Control sperm movements along/release from tubules.

3. Junctions between sustentacular cells create *blood-testis barrier* to prevent antibodies forming in blood from chemical changes in stages forming sperm.

Brain-Testicular loop.

***Gonadotrophin** in Pituitary

↓

Follicle Stimulating & **Lutenizing Hormones**

↓ ↓

Sperm production **Testosterone** from cholesterol in testes.

↓

Some Testosterone converts to **Dihydrotestosterone DHT***

↓

Inhibin from testes inhibits **Gonadotrophin**

↓

Low levels of **Testosterone** stimulate **Gonadotrophin***

ACTH from pituitary stimulates the Adrenal cortex to produce androgens to work in conjunction with testicular hormones. As well as temperature changes, emotion stimulates the adrenal medulla for Adrenalin for sexual performance (and aggressive/defensive responses) linked into the limbic system under sensory stimulus. (*See* The Pituitary. Chap: 3)

Glossary.

Anabolism:...making small molecules into complex ones, (e.g .hormones); (opposite to catabolism.)
Broad Ligament:...a tough fibrous sheet that supports the uterus.
Corpus: *(Latin = body)....* body or mass of specific cells.
Efferent:…transmits impulses away from source.
Electrolyte:…ionises solution to enable it to take an electric current.
Embryo:…developing infant from fertilised egg up to 3rd month.
Epithelium:…outer layer; contains no blood vessels.
Fimbriæ:…fringed edges of fallopian tubes.
Fœtus:…developing child from 3rd month till birth.
Inversion:…tucked up inside.
Involuntary:…not under conscious control.
Meiosis:...distribution of chromosomes. (divide into 2 equal halves.)
Menses:…monthly bleeding in women; release of endometrium (lining of uterus) when fertilization has not taken place.
Oogonia:…primitive female sex cells.
Ovum:…egg…**ova:**…plural.
Seminiferous:…to do with/pertaining to semen.
Spermatazoa:…mature sperm cells which swim towards ripe ova.
Spermatogonia:…stem cells that become sperm cells.
Spermatozoon:…sperm cell with no tail. (tail released once inside ovum.)
Spermogenesis:…production of sperm cells.
Uterus:...womb.
Zygote:… fertilised ovum ie: union of male and female gamete.

Steroid abuse in sport is the use of anabolic steroids to promote bone mass and heavier muscle….
Long term problems:-

- All soft organs and ligaments/muscle attachments remain as original; leads to gross over-working. Muscle attachments tear off; Heart, kidneys, liver etc ‘age’ faster.
- Artificial increase in androgens in the blood eventually *inhibits* the production of androgens by the body itself.
- Cessation of natural testosterone will lead to atrophy of gonads & sterility; development of breast tissue etc in male.
- In female, masculinisation of genitals; decrease in breast tissue, sterility etc.

These will become *irreversible* as natural œstrogen/testosterone production ceases with atrophy of ovaries/testes. Synthetic hormones then need to be taken on a permanent basis. Negative feedback cycle is not possible with this artificial imbalance.

******

Associated Energy Centre for The Ovaries and Testes.

The ovaries lie within the bony pelvic girdle and with the uterus below, are in the energy field of the **Sacral** chakra. This chakra is below the navel and at the back lies the bony 'plate' of the sacrum which is attached to the pelvic girdle. The name **Sacral** chakra comes from it. It is in this pelvic energy field that fertilization, the *function* of both Ovaries and Testes, takes place. The 2nd and 3rd Sacral Nerves coming from the sacrum supply the testes (and penis) although these lie physically in the energy field of the **Root** chakra. The base of the sacrum also enters the **Root** chakra field and this bone is the physical link between the two centres.

Naturally there is a close inter-change between both these lower chakras. The reproductive functions that come *before* and *after* fertilization lie within the **Root** chakra. Thus there is a physical loop effect between the two and therefore a reciprocal energy interchange unifying the two for the strong physical urge for survival.

2nd The Sacral Chakra.

Seat of sexual energy.
Reproductivity/creativity.
Sexual identity.
Gender affiliation/inter-action.
Sensuality.

Positive energy sources:-

- **Physical**:........Normal balanced function of the glands.
  Positive cerebral activity and responses.
- **Metaphysical**: **Reproductive energy.** (man/animal/plant)
  positive/fulfilled **sexual energy**/**lovingness**/**intuition.**

Reproduction, although essential to Man's need for survival and society's continuity, is also accompanied by a variety of emotional needs to have children, some of which come from deep personal issues. Emotional sophistication has also meant that sexual activity has developed considerably outside of reproductive needs. This is a minefield we do not need to enter as we are looking at the sources of negative energy from the anatomy of the reproductive system in everyday circumstances, not extreme conditions.

WHAT

The consequence of imbalance and blockage in this energy centre are:-

Reproductive issues, sexual anxiety,
defensive sense of identity, negative libido.

Survival of the species is the essential function of the Ovaries and Testes. All other survival aspects we have covered up to now are for the survival of the *individual.*

The key anatomical words for this area are:-

- **Ovulation**...............procreation of the species.
- **Testosterone**............sex drive for ejaculation of sperm.

As well as testosterone, **Adrenalin** is a major factor in the reproduction process. In its most basic form Adrenalin is essential to the man for protection of the sperm and for an erection to ejaculate it, and plays its part for both man and woman in the sexual act itself to ensure physical readiness. In our sophisticated world the emotional side is very complex and significant; so the 'emotional' hormone adrenalin plays a major part.

We will begin by looking at the chakra association of the Ovaries. Through their primary functions of procreation, plus the sexual attraction and gender interplay that makes sure it happens, we will look to see what negative energy could impair and impede their energy flow and the centre's circulation which cause problems in this area.

WHY

Sources of negative energy in the Ovaries.

1) Internal Physical.

- Imbalance in hormone production/PMT.
- Menstrual problems/pains.
- Illnesses/conditions/diseases of reproductive system.

Internal Emotional.

- **Self-evaluation:** regarding:-
  - Own female/feminine image/sexual attractiveness/activity.
  - Female gender-play.
  - Female role.
  - As mother.
  - Mothering/ motherhood/pregnancy.
  - Distaste for menstruation.
- Female rôle.
- Gender-play.
- Fear of
  - Childbirth/Motherhood.
  - Sex.
  - Gender Relationships.
- Menstruation/Menopause/changes.
- Sexual problems/issues/anxieties/frustration/lack of sex etc.
- Perceived issues with children/mother/grandmother/motherhood.
- Memories and associations.

- Infertility/issues.
- Sense of failure/guilt.
- Pre-conceptions of status/ 'female' illnesses/menopause.
- Changes in status/role.

Because of the monthly blood loss women have through menstruation, plus the circulation of female androgens in the blood stream for the purposes of pro-creativity, there is a link here with the spleen. This, we have already seen, is the seat of female energy. Problems and issues from the above negative sources will become trapped in the spleen and slow down or block the energy field there also.

Emotional 'blockages' can be readily felt by healers/therapists who deal consciously with the energy system.

As well as our internal sources, sexuality, motherhood and gender pressures are very high profile in modern lives. Thus the sources of relevant external negativity need to be understood also.

External Physical.

- Social conditioning.
- The media in all forms.
- All aspects of Authority.

External Emotional.

Partners/parents/family/friends/associates:-

- Affected by their own issues, *internal* associations and emotional responses causing reaction of negativity in us.
- Chain-reaction from own negativity.
- Children/responsibility.
- Responsibilities in the workplace.
- Matriarchal/Patriarchal influences/pressures.
- Criticism:-of rôle/status/failure to have partner/ children. (from choice or infertility)
- 'old wives tales'.
- Expected & perceived prejudices per above.
- Sexual pressure/manipulation/'emotional blackmail.'

Because fertility and motherhood are so biologically fundamental to women, the sources here are complex and involved. Reproduction, ie: procreativity, and its accompanying parenthood is naturally influenced by female relations: a woman's mother and even grandmother, their issues, and the pressures and problems they too have had, or are having. Their influence is frequently very subtle.

Women need to be aware of all these aspects in understanding themselves in relation to this chakra energy. This would also help both men and women gain a better understanding of female relatives plus help family relationship issues.

We will now look at the sources of negative energy relating to the function of the **Testes** that can and do influence the energy circulation of the **Sacral** chakra in men.

The primary function of the testes is for sperm-production for **fertilization**, which takes place in the fallopian tubes in the female **Sacral** chakra energy. However in the male, the Vas deferens, the tubes that carry the sperm from the testes to the prostate for seminal fluid for ejaculation, and so to the penis, loops up and enters the energy field of the male **Sacral** chakra on its all important journey to initiate fertilization.

Due to the *biological* urge for survival of the species, frequency of the sexual act is paramount for men. With Man's emotional development and social living, the complexities of sexuality and sexual performance are now as important, and an essential part of gender identity and interplay. Fatherhood usually becomes important through established relationships or the birth of a child. For modern men 'parenthood' pressures have now become high profile and a part of current social change.

Sources of negative energy from the Testes.

1) Internal Physical.

- Size of Penis/testicles/performance/stamina.
- 'Impotence'ie: non-erection/infertility/undescended testicles.
- Illnesses/conditions/diseases of reproductive system.

Internal Emotional.

- **Self-evaluation:** regarding:-
  - Own male/masculine image/sexual activity/attractiveness.
  - Male & female gender-play/sexual prowess.
  - Impotence/Infertility/sense of failure/guilt.
  - Male/Father rôle.
  - Fathering/Fatherhood.
  - Son succeeding father issues.
- Male rôle/pre-conceptions/prejudices/expectations.
- Matriarchal/Patriarchal influences/pressures/expectations/demands.
- Gender-play/male status/perceived peer pressure.
- Changes in status/rôle.
- Fear of
  - Sexual prowess/performance/sexual demands etc.
  - Gender relationships/commitment.
  - Parental responsibilities/demands/expectations.
  - Women/criticism from women.
  - Menstruation/menopausal issues.
- Sexual problems/adequacy/anxieties/frustration/lack of sex etc.
- Perceived issues/stresses with children/parents/grandparents.
- Memories and associations.

As all aspects of sexuality and masculinity come under constant pressure for men so understanding sources of external negativity is important.

External Physical.

- Social conditioning/expectations from society, men & women.
- The media in all forms.
- All aspects of Authority.

External Emotional.

Partners/parents/family/friends/peers/associates:-

- Affected by their own issues, *internal* associations and emotional responses causing reaction of negativity in us.
- Chain-reaction from own negativity.
- Children/responsibility.
- Matriarchal/Patriarchal influences/pressures.
- Criticism:- of rôle/status/failure to 'prove manhood'.
- Peer pressure/competition/ridicule etc.
- Sexual pressure/manipulation/'emotional blackmail'.
- Parental demands/expectations:-
  - 'being a son to carry on the name'...
  - 'son to succeed for the father'
  - 'be the father's young self' etc,

Because of the 'parental' aspects of fertility, 'authority', which is ever present in modern life, exerts a strong influence.

For both men and women, sexual success is a very intense pressure. Women are looking for lasting relationships, pressured biologically by their basic nesting/maternal instincts which now has the added concept of social acceptance/success. Men are looking for sexual frequency, urged by their biological need to 'sow their seed widely for distribution' with the added concept of sexual competition/success. Many men and women also feel the need to prove their success to their own gender peers, and/or for personal (Ego) satisfaction. Parenthood is a separate issue in present society because of modern thinking and choices.

We can see that there are many very complex sources of negative energy here so it is not surprising that so many people become strongly focused on this region. Addressing and releasing these issues, therefore, would enable them to discover more life-enhancing experiences through the upper chakras. This would achieve a more light-hearted and enlightened approach to life and relationships as well as discovering more of their capacity for love and lovingness.

The Ovaries and Testes do not make the distinction; emotional issues overlay their function. Loving relationships manage sexual behaviour differently.

A lot of emotional influence comes through the media and advertising. Since they are a large part of modern life, they need to be considered: for example, image and impossible goals/idealised situations, plus negative impressions of family life/sexuality/ parent relationships/authority. Because they are a constant source of information made available and promoted by a huge and diverse industry, these all play their part in both conscious and subconscious views of issues relevant to this important and emotive area of reproduction and sexuality.

As can be seen, the internal and external sources of negativity are highly complex. It is a strong biological, instinctive and emotional area. Influences, impressions and perceptions over these issues are frequently sub-conscious.

A certain amount of conscious negativity is obvious but often becomes so habitual and taken for granted that we don't notice it is happening. Social conditioning plays a large part in this. Consciously or otherwise we don't really notice how much it is a part of our lives and social behaviour.

However when we do, we also suppress our feelings and thoughts on the subject for various reasons. (*See* Throat chakra Chap: 4.p63)

This energy centre has a lot of heavy and complex negative energy to deal with. Testosterone plus adrenalin are a very powerful combination. The bony encirclement of the pelvis does much to contain and localise the energy specific to reproductive and sexual issues.

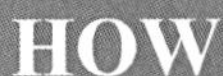

HOW

PHYSICAL CONSEQUENCES

for eg:

- Feeling unmotivated.
- Poor sex-drive.
- Unaccountably tired, 'under the weather'.
- Sexual aggressiveness in some form..(from bickering to violence).
- Low back pain.

- **Women**...prone to:-
- Irregularities/pains/'bad periods', generally unwell at period time
- Weight gain in area of pelvis and thighs.
- **Men**....prone to:-
- Psychological 'impotence'/early/premature ejaculation.

Local conditions or illnesses (will often linger or be recurring.)

Stronger or serious deep issues from all these sources would manifest reproductive and pelvic problems. Local problems, conditions, illnesses and diseases are not only more able to develop, but the healing resources of the body are more impaired also. [If the situations are long-term or extreme or have any element of physical or mental trauma, these issues will be deeply hidden. Aspects of sexuality and parenthood, plus authority issues will affect the individual: being indifferent/in conflict with them, afraid of them, wanting/seeking authority/control, or through an overt authoritative manner etc.]

Any physical manifestations here, or even in other areas of the body, that are *accompanied* by any indications of female/family/parenthood/responsibility issues, sexual problems, feeling sexually unattractive or aggressive, into 'control' and/or authority issues would therefore indicate that:-

Healing/releasing is needed in the pelvic area as well as the site of the condition or illness to give the greatest effect. Attention focused on the **Sacral** chakra can greatly enhance the treatment being given.

Because of the close inter-action of the **Root** chakra and its energy influence on the reproductive organs, healing to this area & chakra would be beneficial also.

All positive thinking is good, but some people can't find or accept a positive aspect to the problems they have. Even to raise them, or wish to reveal them is difficult. If possible consider/suggest that as negative thoughts come up use/try:-

'Positive Distraction Thinking'

Thinking of or doing something unrelated or interesting quickly instead to boost the positive energy to keep negativity at bay.

Strategies for dealing effectively with emotional ties and pain are explored in ***Section 3.*** You will also find more on the nature of energy to help you in the last two sections.

WHAT

This is a very sensitive area because reproduction is so vital and the ovaries have a repeating cycle that needs balanced energy; the **Sacral** chakra cannot retain all the negative energy produced from its functions although it can become seriously blocked. ***Many issues are linked to the Will and Ego*** and involve the **Solar Plexus** chakra too.

The various intensities of Ovarian and Testicular negative emotional energy will **gravitate** or move to the other chakras.

Different aspects will occupy *different* chakras.

- Aspects of confusion/despair will be drawn into the **CROWN** chakra.
- Hopelessness/inability to see ahead will be drawn into the **BROW** chakra.
- Tension from unspoken distress/frustration etc will go to the **THROAT** chakra.
- Sadness/'heartbreak' and Self-pity will be drawn to the **HEART** chakra.
- Anxiety/thwarted will/negative ego will go to the **SOLAR PLEXUS** chakra.
- Fear/anger/hatred/sense of personal inadequacy will descend to the **ROOT** chakra.

Keeping the hormones balanced and the energy flowing freely and vitally through releasing and therapeutic treatments will of course enhance this area for everyday relational and gender interplay as well as help those conditions and illnesses that attract related emotional energy here. Thus massage between couples is very beneficial.

> Here in this chakra, fertilization is prepared for by the ovaries and completed when the sperm enters the ovum in the fallopian tubes. Thus it is in this **Sacral** chakra that the **survival of the species** is physically manifested.

WHY

The sacrum was named thus, ie: '*the sacred bone*' in ancient times.
Fertility was always considered sacred; treated as a 'rite' since it ensured survival. More importantly it ensured the continuation of Man because he held sacred knowledge.
[Part of that sacred knowledge was Man's consciousness that he had been 'created', come *from* something, even somewhere: Man had a future after death and so he buried things with the dead for use in the afterlife. This 'conscious awareness' of himself and fellow man gave 'survival' a further deeply creative importance.]

As a thinking, reasoning being, conscious and 'aware' of his environment and his place in it as well, Modern Man still needs to be conscious of these things in terms of fertility.

> Parenthood involves a degree of control and authority.
> We do need to understand both.
> Without responsibility, Control and Authority are abused.

Parents, in the knowledge that they have given life to their children, sub-consciously perceive it to be a gift. Do we freely give it or do we have requirements of them for it? The parents help create the *body*. The person inside is their own. Like a car with its own driver. During childhood naturally we need to show them, metaphorically, how to 'drive' it properly, safely, with road sense and maintain it adequately.

Adulthood should then be their choice to do as they wish with it and go wherever they choose with it as now they are the qualified driver of their own 'vehicle'.

Letting them do this freely without the parent(s) watching for every bump and scratch and not being a back seat driver is the hardest part of parenthood. We wish their lives to be painless, trouble free and happy and the bodywork kept pristine. This makes us constantly subconsciously concerned over their 'driving'! But the umbilical cord is cut at birth. Do we keep it attached subconsciously, by what we believe about parenthood, perhaps *our habit/need* to continue control, lovingly or otherwise?

It is helpful to bear two things in mind.
One, that cells in the developing embryo and cells in the mother's uterus together create the placenta and umbilical cord.
Two, this partnership of cells *ceases at birth* as the placenta is expelled and the cord severed.
Physically this indicates clearly that life for the child outside the uterus is now separate. We need to be consciously aware of the finality of that separation for the individuality of the child to grow towards full independence. Surely we want them to 'stand on their own two feet'? We want to believe that we do.

We also assume that we do too. Children follow our example; so we need to realise what the patterns are that they will follow and repeat.

Metaphysically this cellular partnership of the placenta/umbilical cord indicates the source of this psychological 'umbilical' attachment which continues the parent/dependent child relationship into and in adulthood with this two way emotional exchange. It also occurs in many non-genetic relationships because this placental connection remains in the psyche. (*See also* p199.)

> If we are attaching someone to us to over-nurture them, then the recipient is taking that nourishment and not using or being allowed to use their own.

We need to ask, how much of our own emotional resources, physical activity, time, attention etc ie: 'nourishment', are we both 'giving' or allowing to be taken and feeding the recipient? What are we actually doing? What level of nourishing are they doing for themselves? (*See also* p221.)

Trusting our grown children to get on with life gives them the right to the experiences that only they can learn from. We need to pass control over to them. Then they can grow and develop freely into the person they wish to be, not the one *we* wish them to be, live like, have what we didn't have and so on. This is to continue parental control and authority past childhood.

This either denies their taking full responsibility for themselves or lets them feel they are not trusted to live fully for themselves. Accepting that this is not a continuing rôle for parents is the hardest part. Parenthood is for life, but it must change, develop and evolve into a purely loving one as we also change, develop and evolve through freely living in *our* own experiences, as we want *our* parents to trust *us*.

Naturally there are two sides to the coin. As the adult offspring of an over-protective or controlling parent, we need to ask the 'how' and 'why' of ourselves about acceptance and dependencies and control cycles. Understanding what is happening and seeing the situation clearly is necessary if any change is to occur. This can be achieved by changing the sub-conscious vibrations within oneself that are holding the situation in place if that is what one chooses. Freedom to be responsible for ourselves is how we develop fully as adults. We need to allow this for ourselves too.

Anatomically this is the area of fertility.
Metaphysically this is the area of responsibility.

My Personal Notes

My Personal Notes

Chapter 8. The Adrenal Glands.

Now we will look at two busy, but very delicate glands, the Adrenals.
They are also known as the Supra (above)-renals (kidneys) as they sit like a little cap on top of each kidney on either side of the pancreas. (*See* **Fig:1.)**
They are well protected: from above by the diaphragm, behind by the large strong muscles of the back and buffered by the larger soft organs of the upper digestive system. They also have a fatty protective coat of 'suet' and are enclosed in a connective tissue capsule. The main hormone Adrenalin, which is familiar to everyone, puts our energy to use in many ways, under both ordinary and extraordinary circumstances. It also inter-relates with the energy functions of the thyroid and the liver and is sent via the **ANS** (*see* Chap: 9) to stimulate most areas of the body, as it is the 'Stress' hormone.

WHAT

Adrenals or Suprarenals.

structure

- 2 layers of soft tissue:-
  Outer cortex & Inner medulla.
- Inner medulla profusely supplied with nerves from *Autonomic Nervous System*………For *fast* action.
- Rich supply of **arterial** blood.

WHY

Endocrine Function.

Hormones produced:-

- **Epinephrine** (Adrenalin) & **Norepinephrine** (non-steroid) for normal Blood Pressure &*'fight or flight'* in emergency etc:
- **Cortico-steroids = Aldosterone,** Antidiuretic **H**ormone
  Cortisol (hydrocortisone) & **Cortisone.**
  Controls *Water metabolism,* & metabolism with Adrenalin.
- **œstrogens** & **androgens.**
  Secondary *sex* hormones.

The hormones produced operate a system of constant checks & balances to maintain homeostasis, stimulating and inhibiting as necessary through negative feedback.

The two layers each have a different structure with specialised and vital functions.
The *outer* layer, the **cortex** secretes into the bloodstream.
The *inner* layer, the **medulla**, works through the nervous system.
A network of capillaries supplies the cortex with blood & lymph.
In the medulla they widen into sinusoids.

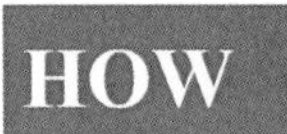

Outer cortex.
Essential to life.
(Life-long hormone replacement if damaged/diseased (eg: Addison's disease.))

- Yellowish, uneven surface.
- *Three* **outer** secretory layers (zones) of **endocrine** tissue producing **cortico-steroids.**

1, *Zona glomularosa*

- Produces *mineral*-corticoids;

these control mineral salts/electrolyte content of blood, mainly **aldosterone:** a hypertensive (*raising blood pressure*) when blood volume drops**;** maintains sodium homeostasis; (normal blood sodium (salt) levels).
(In bleeding; dehydration) stimulates the **kidneys** to retain *sodium* & works in conjunction with:-

- **A**nti**d**iuretic **H**ormone (ADH) from pituitary which stimulates the kidneys to retain *fluid.*
- Promotes excretion of acids in urine; maintains blood pH at 7.35 preventing acidosis.

2, *Zona fasciculate*

Produces *gluco*-corticoids;
these maintain glucose homeostasis:-

- Mainly **cortisol*** (hydrocortisone) & cortisone.
- Accelerate breakdown of proteins into amino acids for liver to convert into glucose.
- Balance carbohydrate & fat catabolism for energy availability.
- Maintain normal blood-pressure by acting with epinephrine.
- Provide resistance to stress…**increasing** blood glucose for energy in fasting, fright, high altitude, bleeding etc.
- **increasing** blood pressure in hæmorrhage etc.
- anti-inflammatory; *counters* response of phagocytosis & release of histamines by *inhibiting* them if too inflammatory.

***Cortisol** stimulates Cortitroph in Pituitary to produce **A**dreno**co**r**t**rophic **h**ormone (**ACTH**) which promotes development and health of cortex and stimulates it to produce and secrete glucocorticoids for utilising glucose.
This in turn stimulates production of epinephrine **(adrenalin)** in the medulla for *everyday* activities of maintaining homeostasis.

3, *Zona reticularis*

Produces *gonado*-corticoids. (sex hormones)

- S*econdary* sex characteristics at puberty.
- Healthy function of reproductive system in adult.
- **œstrogens:** female hormones:
  eg: breasts/genitals/body shape/ovulation.
- **androgens:** male hormones:
  eg: • In males; genitals/body hair, voice pitch, muscle development
  • In females, libido & sexual behaviour, body hair.

Inner medulla

- Reddish due to blood-filled sinusoids.
- **Neuro-secretory** tissue.
- Originates from cells in Sympathetic ganglia. (*See* **ANS** p147)
- Fine plexus;(L = *braid*)of **nerves** surround hormone-producing cells.

Produces 80% **Adrenalin** (epinephrine)
and 20% norepinephrine.

- Both are *neuro*transmitters in **Sympathetic** synapses.(*See* **ANS**)
- Receptors in heart, smooth muscle, glands, internal organs etc stimulate appropriate activity.

Only minimal secretions of adrenal hormones are produced for the specific day-to-day needs of the body that they control and balance.

Everyday functions.

- Help maintain & sustain normal resting blood pressure.
- Low levels stimulates the hypothalamus to release GIH, the **c**orticotropin **i**nhibiting **h**ormone from pituitary into bloodstream to retain normal corticosteroid levels.
- Epinephrine & norepinephrine act as counterbalance to control stress via Negative Feedback mechanism.

The well-known 'fight & flight' response is the one usually associated with Adrenalin. However '*getting an adrenalin rush'* is now a popular modern 'buzz word'; so it is also associated in peoples' minds with emotion of some kind.

Emotion and energy are definitely what adrenalin is about and certainly both are the theme of our investigations of the body and healing. Therefore it is helpful to get a full picture of its remarkable effects when it is in high production. It is stimulated by the Sympathetic Nervous System and counteracted/balanced by the Parasympathetic nervous system which are the major part of the **ANS**; detailed in Chapter 9.

Here we will look at the numerous *unconscious* physical responses that occur under the stimulation of 'stressors', which increase production of adrenalin, and cortico-steroids where more glucose (energy) is needed or being burned. Stressors invariably have emotional as well as physical aspects. A full picture of them is essential for understanding what really does lie behind the much-used word 'Stress'.

HOW

- *Neuro*-secretory tissue in adrenal medulla receives rapid *nerve* impulses from hypothalamus through **ANS**. (short-cut via spinal cord for speed).
- Swift increase of adrenalin & norepinephrine from secretory cells.
- Adrenalin passes freely into sinusoids & into the arterioles.
  1) To **counteract** & **correct** adverse physical changes.
  2) For ***fight*** or ***flight***:-
     Both adrenalin hormones prolong and enhance the effects.

Conditions for increased production.

1).In stress conditions & emergency:-

Physical responses to make best use of energy and energy resources.

- ***Eyes***: dilates pupil/retracts eyelid. (increases vision)
- ***Heart***: increases beat/force of beat to send more oxygen/glucose to muscles; contracts arterioles to increase blood pressure.
- ***Respiration*** increased/dilates bronchioles in lungs to increase oxygen in blood.
- ***Liver***: stimulated to release glucose into blood. (See *glucocorticoids* above)
- ***Spleen*** contracts: more blood carrying glucose/oxygen.
- ***Skeletal muscles***: alerted ; oxygen/glucose/increased blood stimulates motor nerves, muscles work better/counteracts fatigue.
- ***Gall-bladder***: contracts to halt digestive function to save energy.
- ***Intestines***: inhibits absorption; closes sphincters. i.e halts digestion.; as above.
- ***Bladder***: relaxation of bladder wall (detrusor muscle) contraction of floor (trigone) and 'exit' sphincter.
- ***Skin*** Raises hairs: (thus traps air to retain body heat/energy for above needs)

WHY

Conscious:-

Emotional stimulation from cerebrum: fear/anger etc sends immediate *impulses* to the limbic system and hypothalamus and thence to the **ANS** and on to the adrenal medulla.

Unconscious:-

Injury/cold etc; changes due to drop in temp or blood pressure, send *chemical* messages to hypothalamus which sends *impulses* via the **ANS.**

Also involves *conscious* & *subconscious* emotional responses of fear, anxiety etc, so nerve impulses from limbic system stimulate hypothalamic impulses.

2).During labour.

Very high levels of Adrenalin & Norepinephrine released when umbilical cord, placenta & fœtal head compressed during contractions/in birth canal to counteract the physical stress; (more oxygen/glucose needed for muscles and body of both mother & baby).

3) At birth.

- Hormones clear lungs, alter function to air-breathing.
- Promote initial rich blood supply & nutrients for survival out of uterus.

Acute Stressors.

- Physical Injury.
- Exposure/cold.
- Bleeding.
- Anæsthesia.
- Hyp*o*glycæmia. (glucose released from liver)
- Emotional trauma.

5*) On-going* stress conditions.

- Continuation of/*prolonged* acute stressors. (*See above*)
- Stress-related diseases/conditions.
- **Chronic** illness/pain.
- Cancer.
- Obesity.**

Stressors from hormonal imbalance.

- Inflammation of the thyroid. (Often present in Clinical depression.)

Over-activity; prolonged high production of Adrenalin.
- *from* inflammation or
- *causing* impaired function.

- Consistant high production of glucocorticoids.

- **Persistent/prolonged large intake of food especially carbohydrates and sugars, far above normal requirements.
- glucose overload/backed up in the bloodstream waiting to be absorbed by the cells for combustion. (*See* p138)
- Poor exercise therefore low combustion needs.

- High weight gain.
- High blood sugar/diabetes.
- Reduction of gonado-corticoids; loss of libido.

Seratonin counter-acts the Adrenalin fear response in the sympathetic nervous system to restore calm and re-establish homeostasis. Both are neuro-transmitters and therefore work with each other.

Endocrine Connections with weight gain.
The cell absorption capacity of nutrients is set at a norm with some room for extra. This extra simply gets stored when not used. Thus we gain weight.

**Serious over-eating sets up a cycle and puts a strain on the insulin production in the pancreas and especially on the delicate adrenals because of the constant back-up of glucose they have to clear. The over-production of gluco-corticoids needed will eventually impair their function.

- **Adrenals.**
  The overworked adrenals will not be able to produce the full requirement of androgens. Hence the loss of libido. But most importantly, the *reproductive cycle* will be less efficient. Oogenesis can be so disturbed that *polycystic ovary* develops which leads to infertility.
- **Pancreas.**
  The habitual *over-eating, weight gain, high blood sugar, low energy, less activity* cycle of serious obesity creates pressure on all the systems and organs involved. It also invariably leads to Type 2 Diabetes as well. (*See* Glossary)

An impaired energy system has a knock-on effect.

Endocrine glands involved in obesity are:-
- Adrenals.
- Pancreas.
- Pituitary.
- Thyroid.
- Ovaries.
- Testes.

This is without considering the overload to the heart and kidneys and any emotional connections. (*See* **Sacral** & **Root** chakras. Chapters 7 & 8.)

Prolonged over secretion of glucocorticoids *suppresses* the *auto-immune* system.
Adrenals become enlarged as a result of the continuous secretions stimulated by the undiminished physical stressors.
If this becomes **chronic** the *thymus* becomes smaller.
Decreased lymphocytes and allergic responses result.
In conditions of extreme or prolonged agitation or depression, raised metabolic rate increases *thyroid* activity; increased catabolism of body proteins; so there is also continual weight loss with low blood sugar.

Physical and mental stress disturbs the endocrine system. It needs time to recover. It has the resources to do so fully in the short term. Running at under par from continuous emotional and physical stressors impairs our health and energy. On overload all the body's resources become depleted if the endocrine system is taking too much of a beating.

Glossary.

Acidosis:...imbalance in ph of blood (acid/alkali)..acid levels up in Type I Diabetes, (pear-drops on breath) starvation, (anorexia) kidney failure, incomplete metabolism of fat, carbonic acid in blood, in respiratory illnesses or drug abuse. Symptoms are severe and life-threatening.

Arteriole:…small artery.

Blood Pressure:…pressure of blood through main arteries.

Bronchioles:…small airways branching off the bronchi in lungs.

Catabolism:…release of energy into cells from breakdown of fats.

Hypoglycæmia:…Low Blood Sugar Levels.
hyp**o...**Below/Under….. hyp**er..**Above.

Libido:…sex drive.

Phagocytosis:…(Phagocytic (Gk. = 'Cell-Eating') ingestion of bacteria by specialised white cells. (phagocytes.)

Polycystic:...many cysts, (swollen pockets filled with fluid where ova usually ripen.)

Respiration:…exchange of oxygen & carbon dioxide as waste through lungs via blood.

Sinusoids:…small cavity.

Sphincter:…muscular ring in an opening controlling flow of fluids by opening & closing as needed.

Type 2 Diabetes:…The overworked sugar metabolism systems triggers a reduction in the insulin hormone receptors in cell membranes; so Insulin production is thus decreased. Glucose molecules are therefore not able to be diffused into the cell for its metabolism and the glucose therefore remains un-used in the blood. The cells become starved and full function is impaired.

Steroids are fat soluble to readily penetrate the fatty membrane of cells.

******

Associated Energy Centre for The Adrenal Glands.

We have seen the significance of Adrenal activity with its secretions of adrenalin, the 'fight and flight' hormone, and its steroids for sexuality. Both are involved with *survival* which is the principle associated with the **Root** chakra as it is closest to the earth. For this reason, this energy is also the most active and strongest.
When *positive* it creates great motivation and responsibility; when *negative*, inertia, control, dominance and aggression.

The Adrenals are the only organs not actually in the physical region of their energy centre. However, their centrality in the body is necessary because the hormone Adrenalin stimulates *all* parts of the body via the **ANS**, and in particular, needs to prepare so many internal organs for 'fight or flight'. The adrenal cortical secretion (**essential to life,** *see* p124.) of steroids gives constant and essential contact with the ovaries and testes, for their *development* and *function* for *survival* in a continuous physical loop, which also connects the glands to their energy centre, the **Root** chakra.

1st The Root Chakra.
Seat of Survival.

Identity of Self.
Self-preservation.
Defence.
Connection with earth energy.
Initiating growth/development.

Positive energy sources

- **Physical**:........Normal balanced function of the glands.
  Positive cerebral activity and responses.
- **Metaphysical**: **Earth** energy/**Intuition**/**lovingness**/**communication**/**enlightenment**.

Adrenalin is stimulated by the stronger and darker emotions which are the heaviest. Aspects of rooted sexuality for survival generate strong negative emotional energy. Gravity brings these down to the lowest chakra. Also, because this energy can be very dense and even destructive it is appropriate that the very delicate adrenals are not actually in this area. However, their own energy will hold negativity.

WHAT

The consequence of imbalance and blockage in this energy centre are:

Insecurity, out of control, inertia; 'going nowhere' lack of development and growth in life/bitterness.

The *initiation* of fertilization is in the **Root** chakra;

- Sexual responses from Adrenalin.
- Testosterone from the testes for sexual drive and sperm production.
- Sperm via penis and vagina.

The *development* of the fœtus in the uterus begins in the **Root** chakra and also the *selection of the gender gene* from the male chromosomes occurs here.

The key anatomical words for this area are.

- **Sexual development & activity**....Survival of the ***species.***
- **'Fight & Flight'** ....Survival of the ***individual.***

Cortico-steroids from the Adrenals stimulate the production of Testosterone that is so essential for *defence/protector* of the species and energy as *provider/hunter*. This is a very specific energy for survival but, the changes as society developed mean it is used differently as we have become more sophisticated. We now rely on groups of people ie: Institutions, to 'defend', 'protect' and 'provide'. This has left testosterone to be put to other use, eg: work, sport, warfare etc. If it is not used up, (sublimated) it becomes a problem in frustration and aggressive behaviour from plain bad temper, moroseness etc to various states of rage. Allied to deep negative issues it leads to abuse of power.

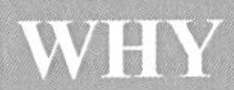

Sources of negative energy. 1)

1) Internal Physical.

- Over-stimulation of Adrenalin/Acute & chronic stress.
- Local conditions/illnesses/diseases.
- Hormonal imbalance eg: PMT, puberty, menopause.
- Steroid abuse leading to artificially high testosterone levels.

Internal Emotional.

- **Self-evaluation**...Insecurity/personal fear.
  Lack of influence/personal & sexual power.
  Low self-concept/self value/self respect.
  Guilt.
- Fear/rational &/or irrational.
- Poor sexual outlet/frigidity/timidity/loneliness.
- Lack of independence/work/finances/physical ability.
- Loss of job/money/material security.
- Life 'going nowhere'. (real & perceived)
- Sense of powerlessness/feeling trapped/resentment.

With women's adrenals producing testosterone for libido and body hair, negative energy can occur from these sources for women also as women take up the male rôle.

Because testosterone is the most active hormonal energy, it responds very readily. Its secondary function is for physical action/reaction for survival.

Increasingly men are sharing the sexual, working & domestic scenes with women. Œstrogen's function remains unchanged, but women are under changing pressures and choices while still intuitively and emotionally involved with motherhood, motherliness and the 'nesting instinct'.

Testosterone's function remains unchanged for hunter/gatherer/progenitor/defender decreed by nature. These biological functions all involve the stronger emotions. Men are being pressured into changing, and are acting against their biological set-up too.

Because *Survival of the individual* dominates modern society, emotional issues are in conflict with conscious & unconscious/instinctive biological pressures.

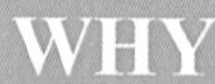

External influences have a great deal of bearing on our survival because 'survival' in all forms is influenced by the society and the people around us. We need partners for procreation, a structure to survive in and emotional support to deal with life as well as experience it fully.

External Physical.

- Physical dangers/threats/hostility/aggressive acts.
- Sexual dangers as per above.
- Media communications as per above.
- Memory associations.

External Emotional.

Partners/family/friends/peers/associates/colleagues

- Affected by their own issues, *internal* associations and emotional responses causing reaction of negativity in us.
- Chain-reaction from our own negativity.
- Criticism. (sexual/work/ambition etc)
- Sexual harassment.
- Bullying of *any* sort; being/feeling bullied.
- Gender issues/expectations at work.
- Threat of job loss.
- Expected & perceived responses to loss of job/money/material security/physical injury/disease.

Because the sex act is stimulated and occurs in this **Root** chakra energy field, aspects of sexual expression and activity will be affected by the negative energy here. Survival and a sense of identity are elements of power; so threats to these will frequently be expressed sexually in some way, either through sex, or hostility/aggression, where both opposite and same gender situations are involved both sexually, personally or at work.

Through either sex or work/money etc either *Power* or *Disempowerment* can become an issue. This varies according to the negative energy trapped here. This is the destructive element of negative energy trapped in the **Root** chakra. This can take shape either/or mentally and physically against the self; eg: withdrawal, suppression of self, self denial etc or against others/institutions in verbal or physical aggression. Positive power empowers the self; negative power is over others or against the self.

HOW

PHYSICAL CONSEQUENCES

for eg:

- General tiredness/no 'get up & go'/poor motivation.
- Self-indulgence/comfort eating (which increase inertia).
- Libido issues; physical & psychological/emotional.
- Body language/voice; signs of anger/hatred/aggressive tension/ underlying fear.
- Lower half of body weight-gain/heaviness.

local conditions or illnesses (will often linger or be recurring).

Stronger or serious deep issues from all these sources could manifest problems in various internal organs due to the distribution of adrenalin, the kidneys for their proximity to the glands themselves and the urinary system also, and the lower bowel. Conditions manifesting low energy are related to issues of disempowerment, especially serious lack of/no energy indicating shut-down. (eg: M.E.)

If the situations are long-term or extreme or have any element of physical or mental trauma they will be both deeply hidden and affect the individual's whole assessment of personal survival and their subsequent related attitude and behaviour, and actions.

Any physical manifestations even in other areas of the body that are *accompanied* by any indications of insecurity, anger or sexual problems would therefore indicate that:-

Healing is needed in the Adrenal/kidney area as well as the site of the condition or illness to give the greatest effect. Attention focused on the **Root** chakra can greatly enhance the treatment being given.

Lovingness and intuition enhance all physical activity so attention to the **Heart** and **Brow** chakra areas will be very helpful.

All positive thinking is good, but some people can't find or accept a positive aspect to the problems they have. Even to raise them, or wish to reveal them is difficult, if possible consider/suggest that as negative thoughts come up use/try:-

'Positive Distraction Thinking'.
Thinking of or doing something pleasurable or interesting quickly instead to boost the positive energy to prevent negative energy building up.

All positive physical activities energise this area at the base of the spine. From happy sexual activity to sporting and physical leisure activities, positive active energy will do much to clear day to day negative energy and inertia of mind and body. The base of the spine can transmit energy right up the back, after all. Healthy energy from the earth is transmitted this way, as well as through the **Root** chakra into the genital organs.

Strategies for dealing effectively with emotional ties and pain are explored in ***Section 3.***

WHAT

Because gravity brings the heaviest and darker negative emotions to this area of the **Root** chakra, the energy circulation here becomes seriously impeded. It cannot retain all the negative energy produced from its functions. Surplus heavy energy then overflows and lodges in the hips, legs and the feet. (*See* Dermatomes Chap: 10)

The various intensities of Adrenal negative emotional energy will have been absorbed by the other chakras.

Different aspects will occupy *different* chakras.

- Aspects of confusion/despair will be drawn into the **CROWN** chakra.
- Hopelessness/inability to see ahead will block the **BROW** chakra.
- Tension from unspoken distress/frustration etc will go to the **THROAT** chakra.
- Sadness/'heartbreak' and Self-pity will be drawn to the **HEART** chakra.
- Anxiety/thwarted will/negative ego will block the **SOLAR PLEXUS** chakra.
- Sexual negativity/frustration etc will be drawn to the **SACRAL** chakra.

Releasing techniques and any therapeutic work on the energy system will do much to alleviate the complex and intense load that this centre and the lower limbs carry. Increasing or restoring the flow will help considerably in improving well-being as well as ensuring healthy and balanced hormonal activity and energy circulation plus help the body's natural healing processes or treatments being given.

Anatomically this area is for Power & Empowerment.
Metaphysically this area is for Power from Earth energy.

Nature in Balance = Self-empowerment.

My Personal Notes

My Personal Notes

Chapter 9. The ANS: Sympathetic and Parasympathetic Systems.

To understand fully the spread of emotional energy, it would be helpful to look now at the nervous system that supplies the internal organs, the *Autonomic Nervous System,* because it is affected and stimulated by the emotions. The **ANS** supplies our internal organs so that they work away busily without our conscious thoughts having to direct it. Looking at this widespread network and its emotional stimuli will indicate why.

Two systems.

- Sympathetic Nervous System.
- Parasympathetic Nervous System.

Work together in a balancing act.
Both are *stimulated by emotion.*

These two systems balance the body's *energy* very effectively between them.

The Sympathetic system is stimulated by the hormone **Adrenalin** (so is very relevant to our studies of the endocrine system) and works *directly* from the adrenal glands to ensure a very rapid response. More than any other reaction, we readily become conscious of the wide variety of physical responses that result from the emotional stimuli that trigger them under stress or 'fight or flight'. Energy is involved; not only physical but mental and emotional energy as well; so there is no doubt of the effects of emotion on the whole body.

We invariably feel exhausted by emotional stress which indicates that the body's energy system is impaired.

The Parasympathetic System, while it acts as a counterbalance to the Sympathetic System for day-to-day function, is also affected by emotion and is stimulated by the senses and pleasurable thoughts and memories.

Through the function of these systems we will see how and why this happens and see how inextricably entwined is the whole body with our emotions.

WHAT

The **Sympathetic** and **Parasympathetic Nervous Systems.**
Together they form the **ANS**, the spontaneous or unconscious nervous system that **regulates** the normal internal activities of the body, (part of but working independently of the **C**entral **N**ervous **S**ystem). They are two distinct but inter-related nerve networks which oppose each other to maintain homeostasis.

Because they are integrated with the **CNS** through the **Hypothalamus** and linked to the **Limbic System,** therefore they are connected to *conscious thought*, *memory* and *emotion.*

WHY

Function.

- The primary function of the **Sympathetic** nervous system initiates the **use** of our energy in normal circumstances.
- The secondary function is to use our energy for *emergency** or *exercise,* and under *emotion.*

- The primary function of the **Parasympathetic** nervous system is to **conserve** our energy in normal circumstances by *ensuring* normal function and rest.
- The secondary function is to *restore* our energy to enable *recovery* from emergency, emotion or exercise.

The hypothalamus regulates the balance of Sympathetic versus Parasympathetic via stimulation and inhibition processes. Receptors from both systems are found in the internal organs giving them a double nerve supply. These act antagonistically to (against) the other to adjust the balance which is constantly fluctuating to accommodate all the internal and external changes in our busy and complex lives. This balancing act maintains homeostasis.

*__Fight__ or __flight__ response.(*see* Chap: 8)

WHERE

Origins.

After receiving information from the main cranial and spinal nerves via the hypothalamus, the ganglia branching off points of these systems follow the midline of the body down the **Spinal Cord.**

Sympathetic System.

22 'chain' ganglia in pairs like beads strung down on either side of Spinal Cord.

- **3 cervical.**
- **4 lumbar.**
- **11 thoracic.**
- **4 sacral.**

Parasympathetic System.

Nuclei in brain stem (source supplying cranial nerves) plus in grey matter in **sacral** area of Spinal Cord.

- **4 cranial.**
- **3 Sacral.**

Physical & Chakra Nerve Origins and Organ Destinations.

Sympathetic....distribution down the length of spinal cord.
Ganglion at the top of the spinal cord...Throat chakra.
The axons *ascend* into Cranium and serve:-

- Iris of eye.
- Nasal mucosal lining.
- Salivary glands.
- Parotid gland.

3 Cervical. (neck)…Throat chakra.

- Smooth muscle of blood vessels in skin.
- Hair follicles.
- Sweat glands.

Thoracic nerves *1-4*...Heart chakra.

- Bronchi.
- Lungs.

Thoracic nerves *5-8*...Heart chakra.

- Liver.
- Adrenals.
- Kidneys.
- Stomach.

Thoracic nerves *9-11*...Solar plexus chakra.

- End of Small intestine.
- Lower Ascending colon.

2 Lumbar Nerves....Sacral chakra.

- Lower Descending colon.
- Bladder.
- Genitals.

Parasympathetic…Cranio-sacral. 4 at top of the spinal cord & 3 at base of cord.
1st and 2nd Cranial nerves.... Throat chakra.
Serve:-

- Salivary glands.
- Lacrimal glands. (tears)
- Iris of eye.

3rd Cranial Nerve. Specific to the **Vagus Nerve.**…Throat chakra.
Serves:-
Base of lungs……..Heart………Liver………Stomach……..Spleen……Pancreas
Small intestine………Kidney…..Large intestine

Sacral Nerves....Root chakra.
Serve:-

- Colon.
- Bladder.
- Genitals.

HOW

From nerve centres (ganglia) there, they pass to efferent *post*ganglionic neurons and to groups of nerve centres called *plexuses* (eg: *solar plexus* behind stomach supplying abdominal viscera) and fan out to the face, internal organs and skin in a vast network of nerves and receptors.

I) Sympathetic.....Utilises energy.
Prepares/sustains body for emergency.

- Impulses move through both synaptically and non-synaptically* via ganglion chains evoking responses in **numerous** organs.
- **Short** fibres from CNS to specific ganglions.

- Mostly stimulated from norepinephrine from Adrenals (*See* p135)
- Some impulses go straight on through* to the medulla of adrenals
- Modified postganglionic cells there are endocrine cells stimulated to produce norepinephrine and adrenalin.
- Neurotransmitters in synapses of the system are mostly norepinephrine and epinephrine* (adrenalin).
- Receptor cells in the blood vessels, skin, heart and viscera etc dilate or constrict the smooth muscle as needed.

- Balances/counters actions of parasympathetic action during normal functions of body for normal use of energy.
- **Dominant mode under emotional stress/physical exertion.**

*this counteracts the parasympathetic slowing & weakening of heart beat & normalises pulse.

WHY

- Stimulation is more widespread in the Sympathetic due to the greater number of initial ganglia and the many efferent fibres fanning out from the post (= after) ganglia that send them on to the receptors in the wide variety of destinations.

- The hormones Norepinephrin and epinephrine from the adrenal glands intensifies the adrenalin effect in the synapses*; so the results last longer than those of the parasympathetic. This is necessary when body is under emotion/exercise/emergency as more energy is needed than during normal conditions.

- Appropriate tissue activities are involuntarily increased with ensuing physiological and conscious responses, emotions and pertinent actions until event passes and parasympathetic system restores balance. The chemical changes when the body is burning up energy at a greatly increased rate as in emergency, triggers the neurotransmitter seratonin as a counter to norepinephrin when the levels are too high.

Seratonin is also produced in the digestive system ready to assist the normalising from the parasympathetic system. This will trigger the seratonin in the brain, ie: in the pineal, limbic system and hypothalamus and together calm the brain and body.

When the adrenalin over-rides seratonin levels from over-stimulation (*see* chronic stressors below) a strong anxiety state occurs and further physical stress ensues stimulating adrenalin production & creating a cycle.

A nerve becomes stronger/more dominant the more it is used....(just as muscles do). **These nerves are more developed/stronger than the parasympathetic nerves in people of a more emotional or 'nervous' disposition or character. Such people also have sensitive or poor digestion.**

'suffers with their nerves' 'lives on their nerves' are well-known but indefinable phrases. Unknowingly, people are right as these people will have stronger *sympathetic* nerves and prone to being under pressure from raised norepinephrine levels exacerbated by hidden fears and negative emotional issues.

There are two main types of receptors in Sympathetic system:
Alpha, for **norepinephrine** (sometimes called noradrenalin) for:-

- Increased rate and strength of heart contraction.*
- Constriction/contraction of blood vessels sphincters, ducts/hair muscles
- Decreasing saliva/Pancreatic processes.

Beta, for **adrenalin (**or **epinephrine)** for:-

- Dilation of blood vessels/bronchioles.
- Relaxing bladder.
- Decreasing peristalsis.

It is because they can be stimulated by strong emotions like anger, excitement, fear etc that these nerves are called Sympathetic.

This Sympathetic system therefore is the *active* side of the **ANS**.
We need now to look at the *passive* side, the Parasympathetic, which calms, rests and restores us both physically and mentally.

HOW

2) Parasympathetic........for energy Manufacture/Conservation.
Restores energy for recovery.

- Tend to serve a specific organ.
- **Long fibres** from nuclei to specific ganglions set nearer organs.

- Dominant system in normal circumstances.
- Reduces heart rate……ensures normal rate and resting rate.
- Deals primarily (75%) with digestive system via **Vagus** nerve.

- Stimulates amylase in saliva to start digestive process.
- Stimulates liver/pancreas/gastric juices and peristalsis in stomach/ intestines to break down nutrients.
- Stimulates absorption of nutrients and elimination of waste.
- Counters/balances sympathetic processes to maintain normal activity. Inhibits sympathetic effects when rest/recovery needed.

WHY

To fulfil function,

- System makes digestion and absorption of nutrients possible in order to supply energy needed for all cellular activity.
- To facilitate the processing of fresh supplies of nutrients, stimulates waste systems, ie: rectum, kidneys, bladder.
- Keeps eyes and mouth moist ie: healthy, for receiving sensory signals to stimulate digestive processes.

The Vagus nerve supplying the digestive system is **only** stimulated under *pleasant* or *pleasurable* sensations, emotions, memories from:-

- Appetizing smell/sight/taste of food.
- Calm, happy/pleasant environment and circumstances etc.

These conditions enable stimulation of digestive juices, efficient digestive functions and waste elimination.

These functions are diminished or *inhibited* and hunger centres (*See* Pituitary Chap: 3) shut down if there is a **lack** of these normal stimuli or under feelings of distress, anxiety, excitement or exertion. This is to conserve energy.

NB. Naturally, people who are ill or recovering from illness and who need extra nourishment, *appetizing* and *suitable food* and very *favourable conditions* are **essential** to ensure:-

a) the flow of digestive juice and food breakdown processes,
b) the proper absorption/elimination processes are working too.

Adverse/poor conditions will inhibit/prevent this!

Main neural actions.

- Dilates coronary blood vessels/genital blood vessels. (sexual stimulation)
- Contracts bladder.
- Constricts bronchioles.
- Relaxes sphincters/ducts.
- Increases peristalsis/saliva/pancreatic processes/tears.

These processes can be over-activated in emotional shock/distress, then chest will tighten and person weeps, or be radically over-activated by what is called *Paradoxical fear*…ie: *terror* or *'no-way-out'* situations, eg: Bowels and bladder open involuntarily.

After exertion, shock, fright, periods of anxiety etc, *restful recovery time* is essential to allow for the parasympathetic normalising and balancing systems to return the body to homeostasis. Re-adjustment after high adrenalin output is very important as the hormone is so responsive to emotion. By understanding this, and acting on this we can help ourselves to proper recovery both in mind and body.

People in whom the parasympathetic nerves are more developed/stronger are unperturbed and placid characters, with good digestions.

Then there are those in whom the systems are relatively equal and who are not too emotional and are quick and alert and active: - ie: what we consider *well-balanced* characters.

It is now possible to see how involved a process there is between our nervous system, emotion and internal bodily functions. Through ***recovery time*** and ***pleasant stimuli*** for the calming processes for mind and body, the parasympathetic system will ensure that the body is making proper use of its nourishment and the energy is kept in balance. Homeostasis will maintain good health and when necessary, enable healing to take place.

Nature's primary urge is to equalize.

******

Glossary.

Antagonistic:…opposing action.
CNS:…**C**entral **N**ervous **S**ystem consists of Brain & Spinal Cord.
Duct:…tube carrying substances out of an organ.
Efferent:…outgoing (nerve).
Ganglion/a:…area of grey matter of un-myelinated fibres.
Inhibit:…prevent.
Plexus:…network of nerve centres with converging and diverging fibres.
Postganglionic:…taking impulses away from a ganglion.
Receptor:…specialised cell a substance binds to.
Sphincter:…ring of muscle opening & closing a natural opening.
Stimuli:…plural of stimulus.
Synaptically:…crossing of impulse over a gap to pass messages from neurone to neurone.

Associated Energy Centres for The ANS.

Just as the internal energy from all organic activity is served by the nerve network of the Sympathetic and Parasympathetic systems of the ANS, so the whole body's energy system is served by the flow created by the inter-connections of the energy centres. Thus the whole body is covered by them both.

As a result, since both nervous systems pass through all seven chakras, the energy from both physical, emotional neural activity (particularly through adrenalin,) and the chakra energy, will all be closely involved. Thus *all* the body's energy will ebb and flow together and the ANS and chakra centres will influence each other accordingly.

Having looked at the anatomy and function of the two systems of the ANS, we can now look at the chakra energy systems involved. Thus we gain a fuller picture of this inter-relationship of emotional and physical energy that motivates, colours and directs our lives and most importantly the state of our health.

The important factor is that the nervous impulses of the **ANS** are *NOT under conscious control* but after an initial *emotional* response, can be *brought under control to a degree* by the conscious brain and 'will-power' as we learn to 'control our emotions' for acceptable behaviour.

This means we have 'reasoned' with ourselves; - to '*supress*' is more to deny the emotion.

Plexuses are very fine internal networks of nerve fibres carrying impulses.

The plexuses that send out the wide spread of nerves that fan out to serve the internal organs start from behind the *heart* serve the upper body/head and *descend* to end at the reproductive organs.

Just as the heart is the central area of the physical body and central to our inter-relationships, so these plexuses are central to the nerve network.

Since energy travels along impulse pathways, then one can see how negative or positive energy can travel to our internal organs from emotions affecting the chakras.

Positive energy stimulates and supports homeostasis.

Negative energy, being heavier, can readily accumulate in the *internal organs* and in the *connective tissue* around them affecting their energy and vitality. This can make homeostasis for balanced healthy activity hard work. Also it can either allow disease to develop and inhibit the healing processes or hold up healing from injury/surgery.

Naturally the ganglia, ie: *the origins* are served by the appropriate chakra which also affect the 'destinations', the organs they serve. In this way they inter-relate with other chakras as the network of nerves innervate the tissues. (*See* **Fig:14.** p160)

Brow & Throat Chakras. Eyes nose and mouth.
(Cervical ganglia) - all part of our *communication* system.

> How the throat constricts when we are heart-sore or heartbroken!

Heart Chakra. Heart and lungs.
Both organs *replenish* the *whole* body with life-giving blood and oxygen, therefore involve all other energy centres too.

Solar Plexus Chakra. Area of *nourishment.*
The central part of the system (thoracic ganglia) serves the digestive system which has responsive areas throughout the whole viscera fanning out from the cœliac or Solar Plexus ganglion from where this region gets it anatomical name.

Sacral & Root Chakras (Lumbar ganglia). Areas of *survival.*
Also area of cleansing; nerves assisting *elimination* of waste; (menstruation/bowels/urine) as much a part of 'survival' as reproduction and also requiring uninhibited physical flow to ensure good health.

> We also need to let go metaphorically of 'waste' from this area too.

We have already seen how much of the body is stimulated neurologically by adrenalin involving energy. The extra physical energy during exertion both in *exercise* and *fight or flight* will also contribute to our positive and negative energy. This will be compounded by the emotions that will accompany it.

By looking at these we can readily appreciate the responses from emotional changes that affect us, from exhilaration to despair in winning and losing, from blushing to 'butterflies', 'crying' to 'cramps', to racing heart from fear, to fancying someone!

Thus all areas of our body respond to our emotions; so the energy generated by these physical reactions will flow into our energy system internally and externally and thus affects ours and others too.

- Aspects of confusion/despair will be drawn into the **CROWN** chakra.
- Hopelessness/inability to see ahead will block the **BROW** chakra.
- Sadness/'heartbreak' and Self-pity will descend to the **HEART** chakra.
- Tension from unspoken distress/frustration will descend to the **THROAT** chakra.
- Anxiety/thwarted will/negative ego, will descend to the **SOLAR PLEXUS** chakra
- Sexual negativity will descend to the **SACRAL** chakra.
- Fear/anger/hatred etc. will descend to the **ROOT** chakra.

The physical reaction through the nerves contracting under tension can readily be felt in the energy centres.

- Tightening of the scalp.
- Tight headache between the eyebrows.
- Constriction of the throat.
- Tight feeling in the chest.
- Tension in the stomach.
- Upper and lower backache.

We are feeling the contraction of the chakras themselves. At times of emotional pain we are vaguely conscious that we are 'closing in on ourselves'. We instinctively feel we want to retreat and keep people out. Thus the appropriate centre (or even several chakras at the same time) our emotional collection area, closes up as a protective measure until such times as we wish to allow people 'in'. Thus we are limiting our social/emotional inter-play by reducing the positive energy that connects us.

Some people prefer to remain like this and are unconsciously keeping most if not all their chakras closed. After all, we talk of people being 'closed up'. The interplay between them and others is limited by this as the emotional energy exchange is diminished.

Thus the physical nerve network and emotional energy act together.

It is important to be aware of this physical consequence to our emotional centres, especially in cases of anger and shouting. This is what is meant by '*verbal abuse*'. This is what we are doing to one another in aggressive or highly charged emotional situations. In particular with regard to children and the elderly or emotionally vulnerable people. We really need to understand what is happening to their systems and their abilities to enjoy or even have relational and social connectedness.

This is why prolonged abuse can be so deeply damaging.

There is little chance of recovery or normalizing their physical-emotional condition. If the body is under-par or ill as well, recovery is diminished too.

******

This inter-connectedness of the internal nervous system and the chakra centres/energy system can only be completed by the peripheral nerves of the body. Once more the source lies in the core of the body, the spinal cord. The spinal sensory nerves branching from it end in the dermatomes, the sensory areas where the nerves end in the skin.

In order to complete this picture, it would be helpful now to take a look at these nerves and the dermatomes in more detail. The next chapter therefore, will start with the spinal nerves and then discover their destination in the skin and the significance to the energy system.

Chapter 10. The Spinal Nerves and the Sensory Dermatomes.

Having looked at the relevant *internal organs* of the energy system exploring the *periphery*, of the body, will enable us to understand how the outer layer is also involved in the energy system. This will complete our look at the autonomous nervous system, its impulses and energy pathways.

We need now to consider briefly the Spinal nerves themselves which branch out from the delicate white fibrous spinal cord. These nerves go on to supply the outer layer of the body with its sensitive network. These are not under conscious control.

There are 31 pairs of these large nerves. They start at the neck and end at the tail bone or coccyx, passing messages up and down the spinal cord. They are grouped according to the area of the body where they originate.

Each nerve has a point of origin at the front and back of the spinal cord from either motor or sensory ganglia there. These fibres then join together to form the main branch of the nerve which passes through openings in the sides of the bony protective vertebra of the spinal column. In this way sensory information ascends and motor descends to and from the brain for interpretation, response and transmission.

The Spinal Nerves.

Cervical: first **eight** pairs, **C1- C8,** serving the neck, throat and arms.

Thoracic: **twelve** pairs of nerves, **T1-T12**that run between the ribs so also known as Intercostal nerves, serving the chest area.

Lumbar: **five** pairs of nerves, **L1- L5,** serving the lower torso.

Sacral: **five** pairs, **S1-S5,** serving the genitals and legs.

Coccygeal nerves: **one** pair which joins with S5 to form a plexus for that area.

****

The periphery of the body is supplied with nerve endings from these 31 pairs of nerves. It is where these nerves end in the skin, *the sensory dermatomes,* that concerns us. Since the periphery of the body is where complementary practitioners apply their treatments, it is only sensible to understand the significance and importance of these nerve ending areas. This will round out our understanding of the anatomy relevant to understanding healing.

Because nerves carry our physical energy in the impulses that are used to keep body and brain informed and functioning, so positive and negative emotional energy will travel into all parts of our body. Being heavier than the electrical impulses in nerves, this gets trapped in the physical tissues of the body.

Our interest here lies in the *point of origin* and their *destination,....*and subsequently, the connection and relationship they have to the chakras.

The *points of origin* of these nerves in the spinal cord relate to the *chakra centres* overlying them. By knowing the *destination* we can then follow the path that positive and negative energy also takes and *interpret the source* of any emotional blockage trapped there in the fascia (connective tissue), just under the skin.

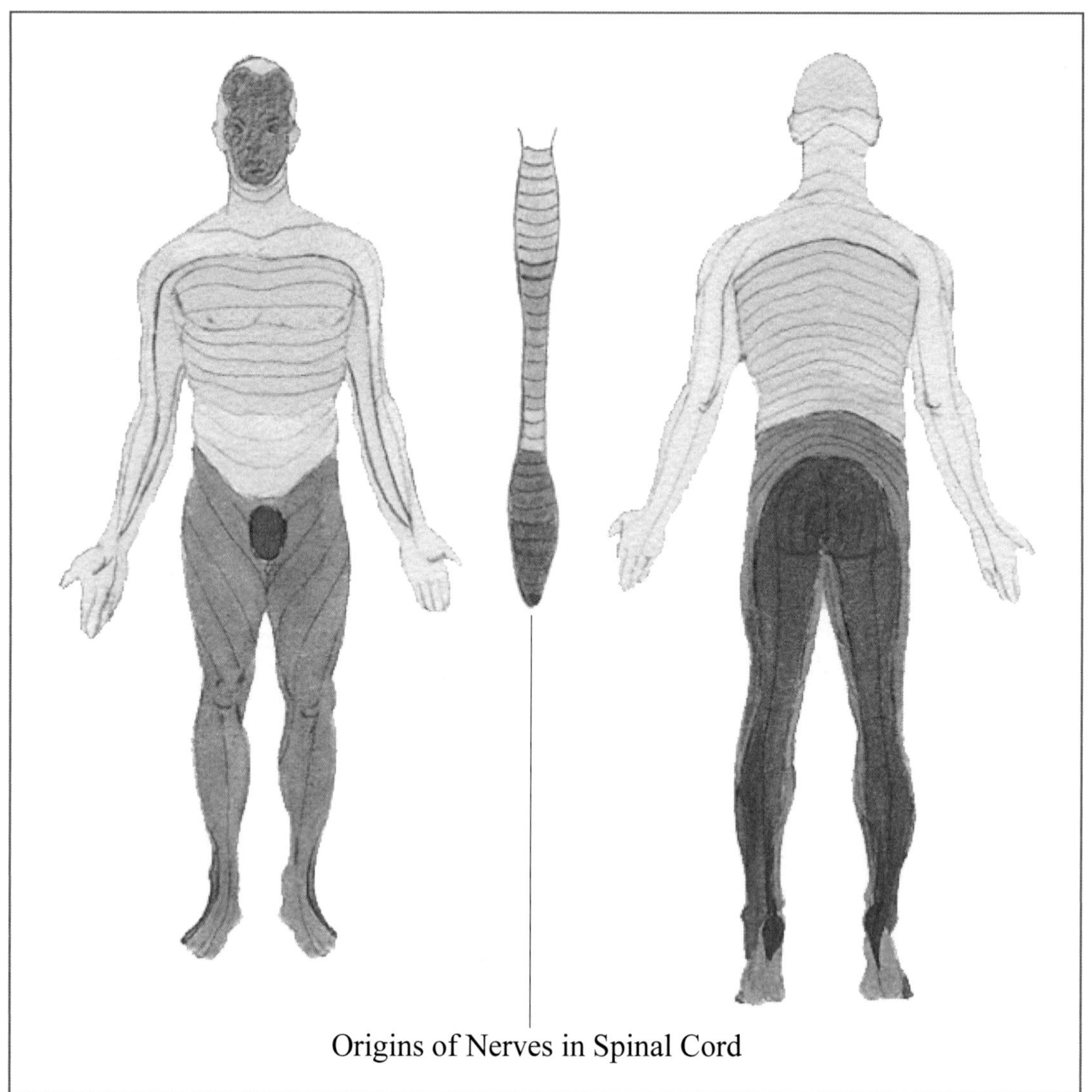

Fig:14. Dermatomes relative to chakras: brow, throat, heart, solar plexus, sacral & root.

By knowing the chakra origins and the destination dermatomes, (*See* pp162-4) we can understand ourselves more fully and realise issues that perhaps had not occurred to us before. This will be invaluable when it comes to interpreting problems and help us work on ourselves through releasing techniques. (*See **Section 3***)

This will also help the practitioner give extra attention to the energy centre or origin area involved when indications arise as s/he works on the body. For example, muscular tension, puffiness, tenderness, sensitivity etc. This is especially helpful in interpreting the limbs.

When interpreting these, the chakra source has to be taken carefully into consideration because the limbs have areas on them from two chakras. Thus the front and back, and sides even, of the arms and legs need to be considered. Separate interpretation is required from what is manifested from the different sources. The arms are influenced by the **heart** and **throat** energy centres and the legs have both **sacral** and **root** chakra origins. Thus for example eczema behind the knee, sides of the legs, or injury to the patella will, therefore, tell a different story.

Importantly too, for the practitioner, the client can focus on issues particular to the chakra if s/he becomes aware of signs of negative energy trapped in and just under the skin as their body is worked on. Releasing these will help in the treatment as well.

Some of the spinal nerves have endings in the muscles. These are somatic (soma = body) and controlled by the central nervous system in the brain and therefore are voluntary motor nerves so not of the **ANS**. However, they will carry emotional energy so that muscles become tense and painful. This can be felt during massage for example. These plus muscles in spasm from injury or cramp will all be felt via the skin. Also any eruptions, bruising or tenderness of any kind in the superficial fascia or on the skin will be the physical response and manifestation of negative energy from emotional problems or issues.

Extra weight gain (ie: laying down further layer(s) of fat under the skin,) invariably indicates related issues or problems specific to the area where the gain(s) have been made. Fat storage is the body's natural protective device for survival; the need for *emotional* protection manifests also in this storing up. Asking oneself '*What do I need protection from or for*?' '*What am I protecting myself against?*' can help in finding the trapped emotional need or demands on you so that you can deal with them. Acknowledgement is half the battle.

To help you with interpretation here are a set of charts for a quick reference to these related issues and the chakra energy centres.

It is important to remember that the *Right* side represents *masculine* energy and the *Left*, feminine, especially where the limbs are concerned. Therefore, this will influence any aspects outlined in the charts.

We experience a great deal with our skin. And each sensation is accompanied by an emotion however slight: all kinds of pleasure, intense joy, tenderness, irritation and even all levels of anger and fear if the skin is painfully hurt. Our brain in receiving all these sensations and emotional reactions, stores them as memories. This enriches our experiences and determines and guides how we live our lives.

******

Interpreting the Dermatomes.

Spinal Nerves	Chakra	Key words	Pertinent Anatomy	Extra key words Positive & Negative
Cervical 6	**Throat**	Communication Expression	Back of head	Tension/vulnerability
			Back of neck	Tension/vulnerability
			Full shoulder area	Tension/responsibility
			Back of arms	Protectiveness
			Back of elbows	Vulnerability
			Sides of arms	Vulnerability
			Hands	Inner conflict
			Front of throat	Grief/hurt/unexpressed feelings
			Upper lymphatics	Detox/infections/PMT swelling

Spinal Nerves	Chakra	Key words	Pertinent Anatomy	Extra key words Positive & Negative
Thoracic 9	**Heart**	Love Lovingness Physical love	Thymus	Auto-immune detox (Un)readiness for adulthood/sexual responsibilities.
			Upper lymphatics	Detoxing/infections/ Fluctuation.
			Lungs	Exchange of life-giving aspects Removal of toxic waste Limitations/Aspects of 'suffocation/stifling.'
			Inner arms/palms Heart. Full term pregnant uterus	Physical contact when embracing, (Un)loved; afraid of; wanting or needing love/giving/receiving love.
			Liver/pancreas/ spleen	Digestion/nourishment/ processing of energy. Mental & physical indigestion/lack of nourishment.
			Kidneys	Filtering/balancing
			Adrenals	Sexuality/fight; flight (preparedness) for Self

Interpreting the Dermatomes

Spinal Nerves	Chakra	Key words	Pertinent Anatomy	Extra key words Positive & Negative
Thoracic 3	**Solar Plexus**	Intellect Will, Ego Launch for ideas	Digestive system	Anxiety (in)ability to nourish self/others/receive nourishment
			Omentum in men (Paunch)	Protective of Will/intellect/ power 'male' identity in society
			Middle back (scapula to waist)	Spinal (moral) support (In)flexibility/Independent physical impetus
			Mid-term pregnant uterus	Development/new beginnings/nurturing

Spinal Nerves	Chakra	Key words	Pertinent Anatomy	Extra key words Positive & Negative
Lumbar 4	**Sacral**	Reproductive Sexual identity Libido Creativity Motivation & mobility	Ovaries	Femaleness/reproduction/ Mother/mothering/ childishness. Lack of any of these aspects.
			Groin	Hernia/weakened power
			Hips	Connect upper to lower back (lack of connectedness/action)
			Lumbar region	(In)flexibility; (holding on to negativity)
			Front & sides of legs & knees	Power for forward action (In)flexibility/can't move on
			Inner thighs	Privacy/vulnerability/ (in)flexibility
			Inner calves	Cramp (cramped/unfulfilled)
			Inner aspect of feet	(In)flexibility/vulnerability/ guilt/preventing movement.
			1st 3 toes	*Right*...Male issues *Left*....Female issues.
			Achilles tendon	Vulnerability/flexibility
			Centre of soles of feet	Verucas/sensitivity to place one is in/at.

Interpreting the Dermatomes

Spinal Nerves	Chakra	Key words	Pertinent Anatomy	Extra key words Positive & Negative
Sacral 5	**Root**	Self image Survival:- (Physical & material/financial) Defensive Aggressive (over)-protective	Genitalia	Passion/outward manifestation of manhood/work power Inner manifestation of womanhood/femininity.
			Non/early pregnant uterus	Preparation/preparedness/awaiting fertility (ideas/creativity etc.)
			Bladder	Cleansing, releasing/retaining
			Sacrum/coccyx	Centre of whole body
			Rectum	Release of solid waste/toxic neg:
			Buttocks	Active power/tension
			Back of thighs	Cramp/vulnerability
			Back of knees	Flexibility/vulnerability
			Back of **Outer** aspect of calves	Cramp/forward movement/ being/feeling 'trapped'
			Ankle bones	(lack of) support/(in)security
			Inner &Outer sides of Soles of feet	Support/arch/correspond to shoulders/responsibility (in)supportable
			Last 2 toes	'pressure'
			Heels & heel pads	Area of Vulnerability from root issues:- *Right*...male *Left*.....female
Coccygeal 1	**Root**	As above	End of tail bone Base of spinal support	Very sensitive Moral fibre (& lack of) Demoralised. Personal power. Powerless/powerlessness/giving away power

We can see how comprehensively the whole body is closely inter-connected. Working on the *whole* energy system, restoring the flow, especially on a regular basis, will help to ensure healthy and balanced hormonal and energy centre activity and naturally greatly aid any healing process. This will maintain good health and state of well-being as well as deal with problems and conditions that arise.

All the systems we have explored follow the **midline of the body**.

- The endocrine glands.
- The Sympathetic & Parasympathetic ganglia.
- The Spinal nerves.
- The energy centres, the chakras.

Thus the most relevant anatomy for the emotions that play so large a part in our lives (and complementary healing practices) is all in the *central core* of the body. From its very centre the vital energy we need radiates out, pervades and encompasses the entire body.

We talk of needing to be, or feeling 'centred'. When we are, it is because the *physical* systems and the *energy* systems are lined up and working well together.

This also applies to balancing the left and right sides of the body since the energy determining both are the opposites, male and female. In harmony they work together, complementing one another. In opposition, weighted one side or the other depending on pressures, issues, problems, negative energy, the body is out of harmony and therefore balance; the core will be being pulled out of line by the polarity from left and right.

How much 'pull' will be determined by the weight.
To which side is determined by the issues involved.

In metaphorical terms, this applies to the male-female partnership, be it personal or in business/work: ie: the person in harmony with the rôle, job or task.

When assessing the condition of the body through its conditions, injuries, illnesses etc, *which* side of the body is therefore often the first clue to the cause(s) and source(s) of negative energy, problems and issues. Any work to relieve the negative weight will naturally help centre the body. Re-aligning the chakras will strengthen the core energy.

All **left**-sided manifestations will be **female-related.** (*See* **Sacral** chakra p120)
- female family/friends involved; children/reproductivity for women.
- female aspects of home/work for both genders.
- women's own negative feelings about/against themselves. (*See* **Brow** chakra p47)

All **Right**-sided manifestations will be **male-related.** (*See* **Root** chakra p140)
- male family/friends involved; sexuality for both genders.
- male aspects of work/home for both genders. (*See* **Solar Plexus** chakra p102)
- men's own negative feelings about/against themselves.

We regularly maintain cars, machinery etc to keep them working well. Even replacement bits are only as good as the engine we put them in to! Why not maintain our own systems to make sure our body works well too?

To help with this there is a whole section on energy itself called *Energy is the Key*.

Once you know all about it, making use of the methods, therapies and skills designed for the energy system will make all the difference to your health and state of mind. And for anyone wishing to work in the field of healing, that of others too. The beauty of it is that is has a knock-on effect as the responses around you become more positive too.

But before we explore more detailed aspects of energy as a functioning part of our lives, we'll have a look first at artificial stimulation to emotion. This plays a considerable part in modern living so needs to be considered.

Then, because it naturally goes hand-in-hand with good health, we'll take a look at the concept of healing itself.

******

Chapter 11. Artificial Stimulation.

To round off what we have covered so far, it would be helpful to look at the artificial stimuli, stimulants and habits of modern society in the light of the energy systems, anatomical systems and their negative feedback already covered.

Understanding what we do to ourselves and why, and giving the body as much help as we can, will ensure that its amazing resources are given full rein to keep us fit to cope with modern living.

We no longer follow nature's biological clock of day and night. With electricity and modern technology we have come to lead artificial lives. The homeostasis which is so essential to good health and a well-functioning body can be affected by this unnatural way of life; but the body has amazing abilities for recovery and adaptation.

But that depends on giving the body good *recovery* time.........so that the balance can be restored.

Sufficient physical activity and a reasonable diet, restful sleep and a positive approach to life does much to give the body this recovery time to ensure balanced organ activity and function and counteract the artificial aspects of modern living.

However, people frequently persist with an adverse situation of artificial stimulation and habits *without* proper recovery time. These will interfere with homeostasis.

- late nights, ...Pineal.
- poor quality food, eating bulky food late at night......Pancreas.
- smoking; drinking ....Lungs, liver, spleen.
- socialising/night-clubbing/pubbing.......................Adrenals.

These are the main areas involved. Physically, these make the body work harder so recovery time is essential.
As well as the physical after-effects, naturally the energy centres are also involved.

- indigestion/poorly digested food.......................**Solar Plexus** chakra.
- a hangover,...**Brow** chakra.
- clogged breathing/smoker's after-taste..................**Throat**/**Heart** chakra.
- tiredness from little/poor quality sleep.................**Crown** chakra.

If a habitual cycle is set up, or there is gross over-indulgence, especially if there are only short intervals between, this will impair the body's ability to recover and prevent natural homeostasis from working properly. Imbalance gets harder to correct the longer it goes on. The work on all the body's systems will be unnecessarily taxing. This invites poor/ill health and will lead to disease.

The whole energy system is involved. The situations from artificial stimulation have a negative after-effect from guilt/regret/feeling physically under par etc, which *adds* to the day-to-day negative issues already there. The whole energy system therefore will be slowed down and sluggish. There is little or no sense of well-being.

We adapt psychologically to feeling tired and unfit so that lack of full recovery mostly goes un-noticed.

The energy system thus remains at a low ebb and the need is felt to 'cheer oneself up' and so an artificial stimulant is sought as a remedy. We do ourselves no favours!

With short intervals and little or no recovery time, the energy level slows down so far that the individual will lose all motivation and invariably turns to self-indulgence and comfort tactics. Breaking this cycle then becomes very difficult.

There are serious social pressures in many fields and these are so much an accepted part of modern life that we have to acknowledge and adapt to them. But awareness and understanding will help to deal with them as long as we are reasonable and moderate in our social activities. Any work on the energy system helps the body recover.

But the mind, through our emotions, is also under pressure and needs recovery time too. Emotions can be artificially stimulated also. As well as positive feelings from laughter, joy and pleasure, the darker feelings are frequently sought as an outlet. Through films and other media output which are designed to manipulate emotions, these can all be 'experienced'. For example:-

- Tense excitement.
- Fear/fright.
- Revulsion.
- Shock horror.
- Overt/Perverse sexual stimulation.

In the short term, these are easily counteracted by the mind and understood as being of the imagination. Intervals of real life and positive living keep the two separate.

If, however, there is persistent and/or prolonged artificial dark emotional stimulation, especially with little or no positive recovery time, the negative effects of over-stimulation will become trapped in the energy system as heavy energy because normalising processes are unable to take place. They then become embedded in the subconscious and attach to the memory and association areas as if experienced and can become part of the person's value system. It will also intensify what has already been experienced and any personal issues as well.

Reality and fantasy/imagination need to be kept separate in the memory.

Both are important and need to be valued and acknowledged as separate needs.

NB Drugs and addictions are a specialised issue therefore not covered here, although the basic factors and principles do apply.

Chapter 12. Understanding Healing.

This short chapter is about healing itself. Before we go on to aspects of the energy centre system (ie: chakra system) and energy itself in the next two sections, there are certain features that need to be explored before either seeking or practising healing therapies. Knowing of them will benefit whatever choices you make for yourself, whether as an individual, practitioner or client.

The key word is:-.....Willingness.
Being willing:-

- To learn about and be honest about yourself.
- To let go of pre-conceived ideas.
- To understand fear.
- To let go of negative 'baggage'.
- To understand yourself, and to help yourself.
- To let treatment take place.
- To receive help and treatment.
- To practise complementary healing/therapies without ego.

Responsibility for healing lies with the individual, practitioner, and client.

- The Healer/Therapist in order to stimulate the body to heal itself.
- The Recipient to enable healing to take place.

The most important attribute to healing is

Empathy.
This is as important as the treatment being offered.
It will enhance any healing practice.
It will improve any relationships.

The individual or the healer/therapist needs, therefore, to learn from herself/himself first. Nobody knows you as well as you do yourself, so you are a perfect source of knowledge. As you have worked through the first section of the anatomy and associated energy centres, you will already have recognised things relevant to yourself.

- Explore and learn about your own issues and sources of negative energy.
- Discover how your own body reacts to trapped emotion.

Once you have started to realise what is happening to your own body, you can even start clearing issues and trapped negative energy for yourself. (*See* Chap: 21) In this way, you, the reader can help yourself to better health, and also understand why and how complementary healing approaches can improve your energy system, your health and well-being as well.

For the practitioner, not only will you be in better health for your healing practice, but also you will realise and understand what is happening to your client's energy system from first-hand knowledge.

This gives the complementary practitioner a unique approach to healing.

Many healer/therapist colleagues are happy to give reciprocal healing sessions to each other. Combined with the understanding of emotional energy and why certain energy centres and areas are blocked will also give them invaluable knowledge, coming as it does from such personal experience from the giving and receiving of treatments.

Healing takes place with positive energy.

Positive emotion and energy can vitalise and activate us both mentally and physically, even make us light-hearted. But often we do not realise that what saps us physically and mentally too is negative emotion and the heavy energy it creates. We feel rotten so that we automatically seek a physical cause…a bug or virus perhaps, '*been overdoing it*' or just '*under the weather*'. Is this familiar? '*I'm all stressed out!*' is a frequent modern cry. We are putting the blame on a hectic life, but again, not on the cause; negative energy.

Although we can change our *attitude* through trying to look on the bright side, that doesn't deal with what's simmering away under the surface. We need to tackle the stuff that is making us tired, low in spirits and pessimistic.

Consciously by:-

- Comprehending negative energy.
- Identifying its sources.
- Releasing internal negative energy.
- Non-absorption of external negative energy.
- Re-energising energy centres.
- Releasing positive internal energy
  1) interiorly through focused clearing.
  2) externally through healing practices.

It is therefore *Conscious Awareness* that effects the first change.
Changing habitual patterns of:-

- Thinking…….(internal).
- Responses…...(internal, regenerating externally).
- Attitudes…….(internal, regenerating externally).

ie:.Releasing oneself from negativity.
Releasing positive energy.
Through knowledge and acknowledgment.
Taking responsibility by working on oneself.

To acknowledge is to hold the knowledge within.

It needs to be more than just thinking it. The *thought* plus *intuition* plus *evaluation* creates the conscious awareness needed to enable the 'knowing the truth of things' within your heart. This is the seat of truth as well as love, for love must go hand in hand with truth.

Being true to yourself helps you to value yourself.

Once you do, loving others is then without requirement for you have no need to feel unworthy and needing proof of being loved. Clearing negative thinking against yourself keeps the balance between knowing why and judgment.

Working consciously on having a positive attitude as a way of life is a good habit to develop. Becoming 'consciously aware' of any negative thinking and changing it with the aim of helping to shift your own perspective on things immediately helps your energy system by reducing or even eliminating, the emotional response.

Having seen how the body uses its systems to maintain and sustain its own equilibrium, it is important to give it every chance to do so by supporting its efforts.

Trying for *emotional equilibrium* is one of the
best ways to help *physical equilibrium.*

The most frequent word used in conjunction with complementary healing approaches is '*relaxation*'. This reduces physical and mental stress, the *very help* the body needs in order to restore that essential equilibrium to combat the abnormalities that lead to illness and disease. How necessary is that? In conditions of homeostasis and dynamic energy the body is fully capable of this. However, relaxation has become linked largely with 'chilling out' with indulgences such as pampering, or alcohol for example. Its significance to healing has become lost.

It is to be hoped that by understanding the body in terms of emotion and negative energy, the true implication of the word 'relaxation' will become recognized plus a better appreciation of its part in approaches to energy restoration.

******

My Personal Notes

My Personal Notes

Section 2. The Energy Centres.

This section is to help to clarify the energy centres widely known and accepted as chakras. It is a Sanskrit word for 'Wheel of energy' because these centres which aid the circulation of our energy were identified and worked on in ancient India. We will look at the seven main chakras we have covered in Section 1 in more detail. This is a further exploration of the centres themselves, what they are about, how and why they work and the energy flow that they circulate.

The midline of the body is the focus of all that we are exploring and the chakra system plays a highly significant part in it. Although there are also lines of energy which run down and across the body called meridians which are worked on by specific therapies, we are concerned here with the major rôle of the chakras and their system. Naturally the meridians and chakras work as a whole; their condition is inter-related, therefore co-dependent. Any work to clear trapped energy around organs helps the flow along the meridians. However, the condition and circulating energy of the centres determines that of the whole body through the quality of the mental and physical energy at its core.

We will also look at the why and how of the colours associated with these chakras and explore the significance of their vibrations. The colours shown and described here are of course when the energy is flowing completely freely. What the centres should look like in fact! The illustrations here, however, are only diagrammatic and show the chakra colours and shape in their ideal state. The colour within each fully vibrating chakra will be well-defined because the energy is most focused there; but naturally since it is energy that flows through them, the colours will overlap or diffuse slightly into the ones on either side through the areas between them, because it is a moving force. We'll see also that the centres themselves interact with one another to balance and harmonise our energy.

Daily fluctuations and any trapped negative energy will naturally create differences and distortions in the colour range in each individual. The shape can also be altered by the amount of negative energy trapped, pressuring or influencing the centre on a day to day basis. These can always be improved by the work we are willing to do to help ourselves on positivity and letting go of dense areas of trapped emotions. The whole energy system being in constant movement will be working to keep as much of the chakra energy moving even if it is blocked in the centre. Thus, all positive physical as well as mental activity can do much to stimulate this by maintaining vitality. Conscious awareness of this can be achieved once we know what and why the centres and their system are all about.

Knowing about the chakra energy centres also helps to understand those techniques designed for therapists to clear, align and energise them. Since these and indeed all hands-on treatments play their part in freeing up the energy system, understanding the chakra system makes it is easier to see that help is available in a practical form from practitioners of these healing approaches.

Chakras in Relation to Endocrine Glands.

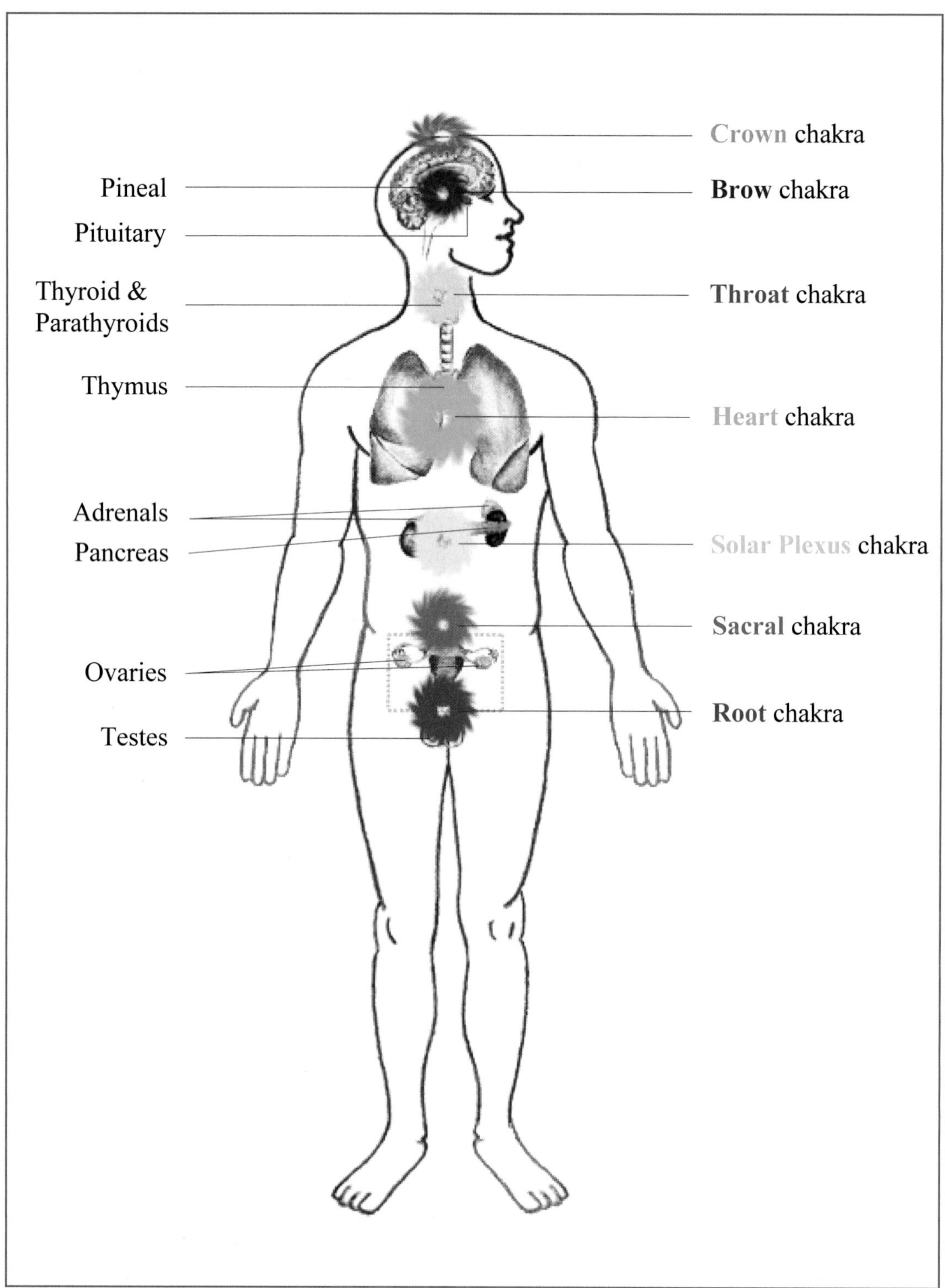

Fig:15. The 7 wheel-like energy centres down the core of the body.

Chapter 13. Chakras, wheels of energy.

As with all living things, we produce an energy field around us and within us. It flows through and around the body and down it from head to foot. It permeates the whole body. Due to the internal workings of the body, energy lines known as meridian lines flow down and across the body and pulses of energy from the organs create intersections where the energy flow crosses.

Having explored the endocrine systems and inter-related organs,, it can be seen that both physical and emotional energy are generated within the core of the body. As it radiates through it and outwards, so the energy field is created.

The *chakras* are wheels of energy at the 7 major intersections as the flows cross.
They are at points where emotional energy is most concentrated.
The meridian lines following internal activity are the onward flow of our energy and the pressure points used are at the minor intersections of energy crossings.

Negativity trapped in particular organs or areas block these points and can be treated by both pressure therapies and chakra clearing techniques.

WHY

These wheels of energy at the front and back are the mainstay of this energy system. They form a channel of energy from **root** to **crown** and the chakras gently rotate internally to draw the energy upwards to the **crown** chakra so that all the active energy enters the passive higher chakras to:-

- Give impetus to initiate aspirations of the upper chakras.
- Be modified by the calmer energy of the upper chakras.

Balanced physical energy from the deep internal organic activity becomes part of the internal rotating energy flowing through the chakra channel and is circulated to add to the external layers.

The Chakras have three main purposes:-

- To rotate energy.
  Internally as above.
  Externally they act as a kind of roundabout at the back and front to keep the energy flowing around and down the body.
  Free flowing energy helps to prevent surface negative energy from our emotional systems from collecting and blocking the flow. The better the flow the more it disperses. All positive energy boosts this energy flow.
- To act as a point of tension to maintain the flow's shape and structure.
- To counter gravity to enable the flow of energy across the body.

The chakras, therefore, are part of a whole connected system of our personal energy force, our Life Force, that *envelopes* and *pervades* our whole body. Thus we can see why and how the chakras are linked to one another.

HOW

Happy and positive cerebral and physical activity charges the energy field with lively energy. Energy generated internally is moved through the system by being constantly drawn towards the externally circulating energy. Meanwhile as the rotating energy flows up through the **Crown** chakra, gravity enables it to flow down over the surface of the body constantly to refresh it. This constant refreshment is to keep our energy at its optimum.

By understanding even the basics of this complex system and bringing our conscious awareness to it, we can also help ourselves to a look after this vital life-force.

The flow of this energy system through physical and emotional vitality maintains and sustains the energy levels that determine our *health* and *quality of life*.

Any reduction or diminishing of this energy:-

- Reduces motivation, both mental and physical.
- Creates vulnerability to ill-health.
- Is present with illness, varying with differing degrees of ill-health or illness/disease.

The chakras and meridian lines maintain the form and shape of the energy system which closely follows the contours of the body. It is essential to health and well-being that this is kept at an optimum. Restoring and maintaining this is the work of positive energy and healing.

It is this energy system, therefore, that complementary healing works on to improve or restore through the non-invasive methods practised. Most are consciously for the purpose of enabling the energy to flow freely but any 'hands on' healing activity works on this system and the energy flow.

The condition of the Meridian lines running down the body will naturally relate to the rotation of the chakras. These lines of energy pulses are affected by the energy of the internal organs and outer layers of the body whose condition influences the whole energy system.

It is the endings of these meridian lines in the soles of the feet and the palms of the hands that are worked on in various pressure treatments.
(Eg: reflexology, massage etc)

This whole network of interactive energy will therefore respond to the body's condition.

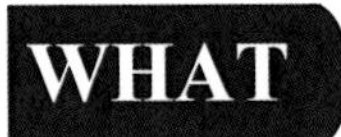

The energy system comprises.

The energy system comprises.

- *Internal* sources.

1. Physical energy from the body's metabolism.
2. Emotional energy from the brain's memory processes.
3. Personality of the individual. ie: mental energy.

- *External* sources.

1. The Aura.
2. All external energy from all living forces from the world about us (man, animals, plants, Earth, minerals.) inter-relates with ours.

In *metaphysical* terms, the **Aura** around each individual, which is made up of several layers of etheric energy, surrounds and contains this energy field and reflects the condition of the energy system.

This is the 'space' we occupy; the one we say we 'don't want invaded.'

The energy system and its auric field responds on the subtle planes of the conscious and subconscious in our encounters and relationships with all living things through both positive and negative energy.

HOW

Persistent negative energy.

Trapped in the physical body, it manifests itself in physical ailments and conditions.

Trapped in the energy system and auric field, negative energy is transmitted to:-

- The physical body.
- *The negative energy in other living things* (or even trapped in places). via the subtle vibrations from both the conscious and subconscious.

- Negative energy attracts negative energy from external sources created by:
  - Response to *our* transmitted negative energy.
  - Negative energy generated by others.

See *Section 3* for further info:

WHY

It is possible now to see why and how the energy system becomes sluggish when negative energy invades or blocks a chakra. This effectively slows down or impedes the rotation of the energy centres (both through the internal channel and/or the outer layers.) This induces the feeling of always feeling tired or 'never having enough energy' for no particular reason. If the root chakra where the darkest energy gets trapped is densely blocked, the system is going to have a hard time of it.

Freely rotating energy through the channel from the **Root** through the body to the **Crown** chakra is needed therefore to keep the body at optimum health. Any work to clear charges of negative energy from the front and back of the chakra energy centres will naturally enhance this flow. The physical body, as well as the external layers that make up the aura of energy around it, is re-charged by fresh positive energy flowing through the chakra channel.

> Energy from the Earth* is drawn up into the **Root chakra.**
> Spiritual or Higher Thought energy is drawn to the **Crown chakra** and circulates through the chakra channel and thus the whole energy system.
> This connection of the body to Higher Thought or Spirituality as energy flows freely is **essential to balance *physical* needs with reason and conscience.**

***The condition of our planet, therefore, is relevant to our own health and well-being. Any abuse of it affects us all.**

******

The flowing quality of positive energy enabling the chakras to maintain the circulation, however, enhances not only our own system but also that of others.

> The quality of harmony of the energy system reacts with the state of the energy system(s) it encounters. This is why we are 'in harmony' with someone or there is 'discord' or irritation between people.

Conscious awareness of the inter-action and reaction of the energy systems of those around us will help us to develop relationships and make encounters with others better.

While there is an instinctive understanding in us for personal boundaries, allowing for changes in the energy fields of ourselves and others and the need for these to be readjusted will reduce conflict and irritable feelings.

Relationships will be enhanced by understanding this need for re-adjustment and giving appropriate 'space' and time for ourselves and others. This will also prevent your own energy field from being disturbed if you encounter disharmony or negativity in another's.

Knowing what the chakras and energy system are all about will enable you to work on them for yourself, encouraging your own positive energy and perhaps clearing trapped negative energy yourself and/or through the help of practitioners in this field.

It is the energy field that responds to the energy field of crystals and therefore they can be used to clear & balance it.

For the healer or therapist also, more awareness of the connections **they** make **within** themselves will enhance their approach to their chosen field(s).

This knowledge and awareness will help in their own preparedness, creating a oneness between *Healing Channeller* and *healing energy,* the *Therapist* and *therapy*, that will benefit both practitioner and client. In this way the *practise* of any method is **holistic** in itself.

The whole body of the healer/therapist is involved

Conscious awareness for the purpose of healing as a chosen way involves:-

The knowledge acquired in training and experience..............**Crown** chakra.

The perception and intuition involved with the client.............**Brow** chakra.

The use of the hands..**Throat** chakra.

The willingness to help and learn through healing practice.......**Heart** chakra.

The physical actions of the therapy itself.........The **three lower active** chakras.

By bringing a conscious focus on the involvement of their own chakras, practitioners will become attuned to their chosen method in a vibrant and positive way that will enliven their own energy systems before any session.

Additional benefit can be gained by practitioners themselves through understanding, clearing and harmonizing their own energy system. What an enormous benefit there will be in their own health and well-being and, as a very natural consequence, any complementary healing that they do for others.

Thus our energy system affects our body, mind, emotions and ultimately the Higher Self or Soul.

The Energy Flow Through the 7 Main Chakras

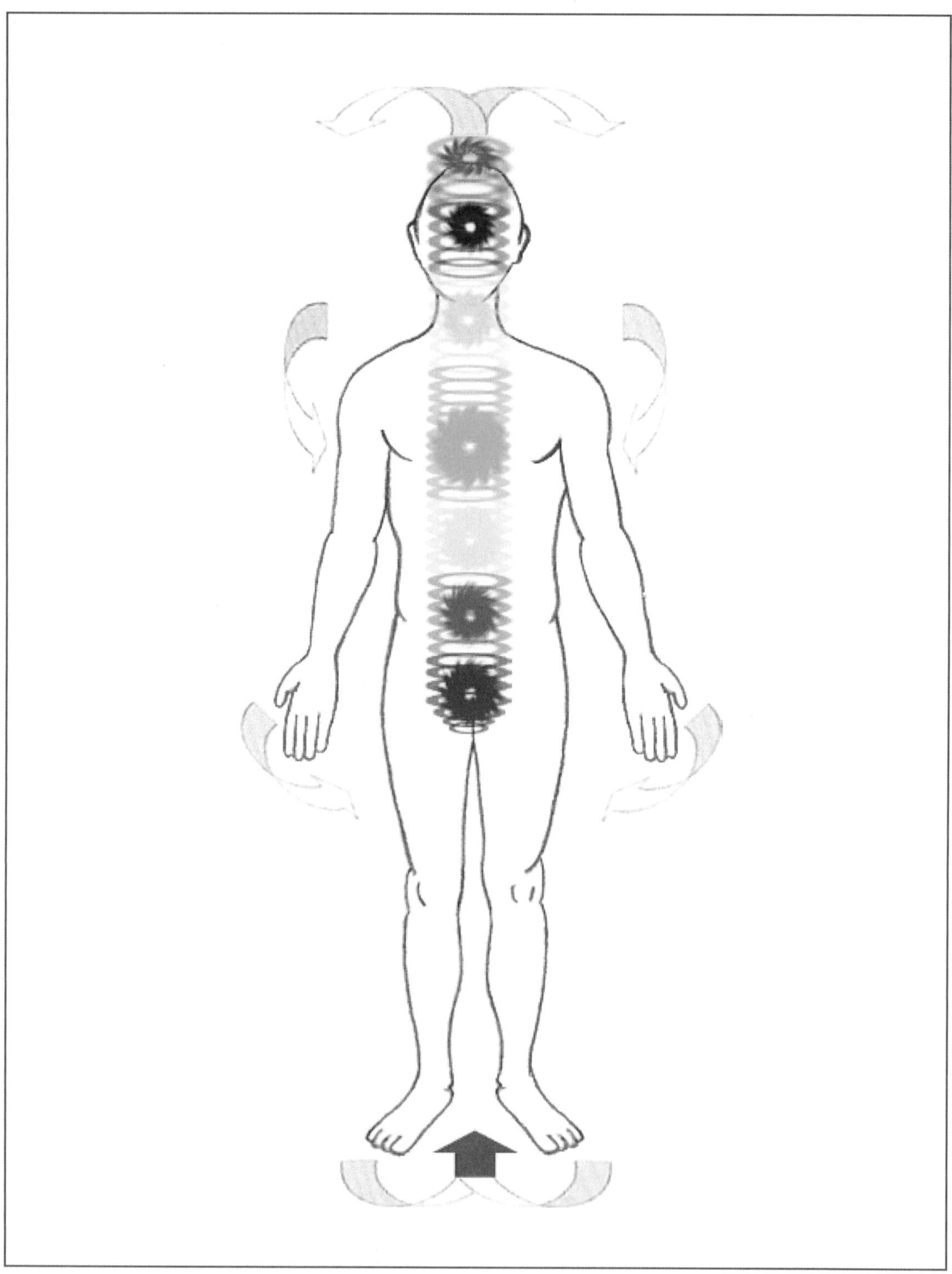

Fig:16. Energy spiraling through the chakras and flowing round the body in a contiuous vital field. Energy from the Earth joins this flow too.

Chapter 14. The Chakra Colours.

The chakras are recognised by the colours of the rainbow. Here we will look at *why.*

The energy in each centre vibrates to the frequency of each of these colours and combine to create an energy cycle. When vibrating freely throughout the upper and lower chakras they create a 'whole' system of one colour. They are also connected in an inter-relationship through their range which we will also look at to discover why.

We will look at this in detail through the colours,their position and their relationships.

Root	Sacral	Solar Plexus	Heart	Throat	Brow	Crown
red	orange	yellow	green/pink	blue	indigo	violet

The 3 *upper* chakras are the *cool* end of the spectrum as they are the *passive* and *spiritual* chakras nearest the ether.
The 3 *lower* chakra colours are the *warm to hot* end of the spectrum as they are the physical *active* chakras nearest the earth.

The heart is the fulcrum and the central colour, Green.

When these 7 colours are combined they make virtual **white**. This is the colour considered for the Higher Self or soul, where all the freely-flowing, positive, combined energy unified into *one* colour, rises to just above the body.

The 3 upper chakras: the higher self or spiritual **Passive** chakras, 'guide' our *physical* selves to aspire to the best possible state of living and being.

7th Crown.
Seat of higher thought/spirituality/spiritual aspiration
Positive thinking

6th Brow. (Ajner))
Seat of feminine principle
(feminine principle/element for both genders) Intuition

5th Throat.
Seat of Communication/Expression
voice and hands (with other chakras defines 'body language')

The cool range of the passive chakras.

The **Blue** of the **Throat chakra** is the coolest primary energy colour and is the seat of the vocal cords and our most (to human beings, primary) expressive area. For the best communication we need to be cool, calm and collected; so we need 'quiet' energy here.

Indigo has a basis of cool spiritual blue energy, but some green from the heart (love) and some red from the root (instinct/survival) are drawn up to this area as the energy combination necessary for the **intuition** of the **Brow chakra**. Thus in our brain, the very control centre, the energies of the body, the heart and intuitive mind are combined and connected for discernment and understanding of ourselves and life's experiences.

Violet unifies both **earth** and **spirit/higher thought** energies in the **Crown chakra.** The blue spiritual energy draws up some red active energy from the root chakra and therefore is softened as it approaches and combines with the highest spiritual white energy of the Higher Self or soul. Here in the **Crown**, therefore, *mind*, *body* and *spirit* are **unified.**

Green is the colour we most associate with our living planet. It is the colour of growth. When we see the earth is green, we feel nourished and that all is well. It is at the heart of our physical lives. Metaphysically the heart is the seat of emotional and higher principle growth. As humans we have developed the capacity for unconditional and/or spiritual love which elevates physical love to higher aspiration. Thus red and white combine to form pink energy when the heart is compassionate.

4th Heart.

Central chakra containing *passive* and *active* energy;
Seat of Love….2 elements
Active……*physical* feelings/expressions of love.

Passive …Unconditional/spiritual lovingness.

As the heart is central to the human condition, so it is to the energy system and the chakra energy centres

The **Heart chakra** as the centre or fulcrum has *both* **active** and **passive** energy and aspects.

Green can be either cooler, mixed with *blue* from passive/spiritual influences from above, or

Warmer, mixed with *yellow* from active. influences from below

Pink is the softest mix of red and white from either *end.*

The *physical* balanced by *higher thought/soul* = *compassion*

The 3 Lower chakras; the physical **Active** chakras determine action of the physical body but also give impetus to the *passive spiritual* chakras to initiate aspirations and outcomes of higher thought.

3rd Solar Plexus.
Seat of Male principle.
Intellect, will, ego.

2nd Sacral.
Seat of sexual energy/reproductivity/creativity.

1st Root.
Seat of survival/earth energy/growth.

.

The warm range of the active chakras.

The yellow energy of the Solar plexus naturally is the colour of the **sun**.

The **red** energy of the **Root chakra** is the warmest as it is nearest the **earth** energy and the **magma heart** of the earth.

The **orange** energy of the Sacral **chakra** is a mix of the two as **reproductivity** is a mix of *growth and development*, from the **sun** and **earth**, elements which are nature's own.

Because the chakra energies are not static, the colours within move and fluctuate from interactive energy and the state of mental and physical energy of the individual.

When they are flowing at their optimum, the chakras keep their aspect of the spectrum separate, as in the rainbow. Due to the fluctuations in each persons' energy and the extent of any shadows or blocks, so the colours will dim or glow. This is reflected in the aura. When there is interaction between the chakras, either positive or negative, the colours and tones will absorb a little from those involved. This is also reflected in the aura.

We know that visible colours affect us psychologically. The colours in the energy system work on the subconscious level, influenced by the energy from the source behind them.
This plays its part in our inter-activity, inter-relating and even in parting.

Auras can be photographed. The colours revealed depend on aspects of mood, health and energy of the person at the given time. Some intuitive people and psychics can feel or even see auras readily, sometimes in great detail or specific circumstances. During treatments many people have seen these colours involuntarily in their mind's eye.

The Physical and Metaphysical Nature of the Seven Chakras

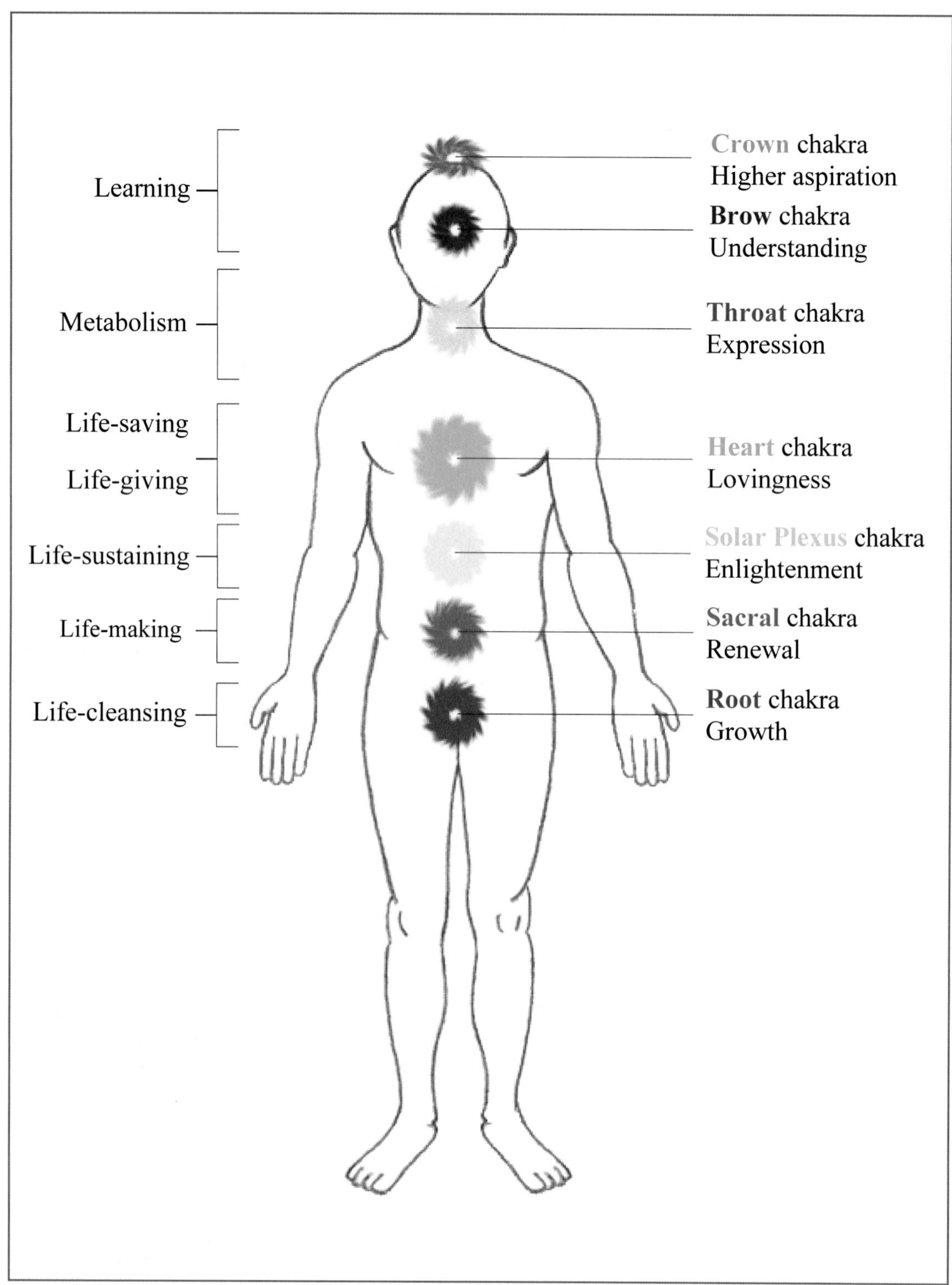

Fig:17. The 7 rotating chakras, where the energy is at its most potent.

Chapter 15. Inter-Active Chakra Groups.

We will now look at inter-relationships within the chakras.

Within the chakra system, there are significant groups. Two main ones are the three upper and three lower. Both groups have an *energy principle*; the upper, the female, the lower, the male. Their position is significant.
- In the upper passive (spiritual/etheric) three, the *female principle* is the *balance* point. None dominate but are *integrated* by the harmony of the three.
- In the active lower three, the *male principle* dominates.
This is designed to *manage* or manifest the activity of the other two.

Both groups are then balanced by the Heart chakra and integrated together by free-flowing chakra energy. Its condition determines the quality of their functions.

In physical terms this is both significant and important too. Each man and woman has these two principles. Both are valuable in all spheres of life. So also are those aspects of the heart in what we do, and also how, in order to balance and integrate them.

Other groups occur when there is a particular need or focus on an energy centre. The chakras on either side of the one that is central to the group, effectively balance and enhance it when the energy is positive and flowing. Because they influence the central chakra, negativity trapped within them will have an effect also. Understanding these groups and the pathways created when they come in to play will help in making good use of chakra energy and in interpreting the body in both positive and negative terms for understanding yourself and others.

Upper Higher Self or Spiritual chakra groups.

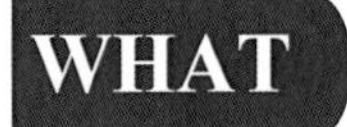

Throat Chakra group.

Brow chakra; above.
Throat; central.
Heart chakra; below.

This is the most significant group because the human voice is our most obvious and immediate form of communication. We consider it our primary source for relationships of all kinds and any knowledge of an individual that we meet.

Both *physically* and *metaphysically* the throat is the area of
- social contact/expression,
- growth,
- balance.

Anatomically through the vocal chords and thyroid/parathyroid for metabolism/blood calcium. (For skeleton & muscle tone) (*see* Chap: 4, p58)

WHY

Throat lies *equidistant* between Heart & **Brow** chakras.
The Throat chakra is a very significant & important chakra; frequently overlooked.

The Throat chakra is the seat of 1) *conscious communication.*
2) *subconscious vibration.*

- Only chakra *not* in a substantial cavity; therefore the most vulnerable.
- Lies at physical connection between 'body' and 'head'.
- It responds *physically* to both conscious & subconscious influences.
- Links with active lower chakras due to physical responses.
- The **Brow** & Heart chakras on either side emit *unconscious passive* vibrations from the subconscious which will be taken up by Throat chakra.

The Throat is the most sensitive to emotion.

Manifests physically:-

- In the voice.
- In the neck & throat muscles even when not speaking.
- In the hands/shoulders/arms.
- Overload goes to lower chakras & determines body-language.*

HOW

Intuition from brow and either *compassion* or *love/caring/consideration,* act as guides to speech in both words and sound; we are clear and moderate in what we say; voice is comfortable, pleasant-sounding, all inviting positive response.
Lack of flow from either can inhibit speech which invites negative response; eg:

- Wrong words, defensiveness.
- Sound of voice is harsh, overloud, submissive, argumentative etc.
- Generally allows inappropriate communication.

It is during rehearsals that singers and actors bring these three chakras into harmony.

WHAT

Solar plexus **chakra** group….**Centre** of the **torso**

Throat and Heart; **2 passive** chakras above.
Solar plexus.
Sacral and **Root**; **2 active** chakras below.

WHY

Solar Plexus; Seat of solar light - natural entry centre for the clarifying light of the sun.

Physically and ***metaphysically***:-
Solar light is *creative energy*. (It is after all the earth's source for growth and energy.) The solar plexus itself is a large network of nerves, sending and receiving information, tucked behind the stomach, source of our ingested food.

Brings **clarity of knowledge** & **truth** on to the **Will** & **intellect.**
These make for personal growth and development in the home/school/workplace etc through:-
- discernment.
- clarity of assessment.
- action to be taken.

> The stronger the sunlight, how much more is revealed!

WHAT

Physically.
Makes nourishment available for absorption from selective activities of stomach, pancreas, liver.
Metaphysically we are nourished by best use of thinking, reasoning, and digesting knowledge to gain understanding.

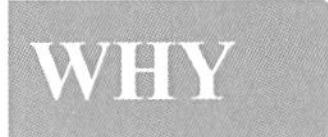

Quality of body.
1) Determines physical state of body through the food we eat and use made of its nutrients to sustain and nourish the body physical.
Metaphysically.
Ideas and knowledge taken into the mind.
Worked on by intellect and will from conscious brain for absorption into mental system memory & the subconscious.
Quality of life.
2) Solar energy from chakra for development and expansion.
Solar light is enabler/energiser for lower physical energy, giving impetus to upper passive chakras for mental and spiritual, or higher, 'growth'.

Influences are:-
Passive energy.
Throat & **Heart** chakras.
Active energy.
Sacral & **Root** chakras.

HOW

Consciously brings thinking into central Heart chakra.
Conscious awareness from focus of Heart chakra on ideas and knowledge enables *comprehension.*

Free-flowing energy between these chakras links **communication** and **higher thought** with **physical** energy for *thinking* and *doing* to better advantage.
Heart balances *ideas/will/ego*; determines quality of *verbal expression* of ideas/will/ego.

If there is negative energy blocking this group pathway, we feel we can't 'get it together' for some reason; our thinking is either all over the place or is very negative about what we are trying to get across. By drawing the thinking into the heart chakra energy, we can centre ourselves and function better.

WHAT

Central Heart chakra group.
In this group, the Heart chakra has a passive and an active chakra on either side. The Heart acts as a balance between both elements and brings its influence to any communication involving the Will and Ego.

Passive energy.
Throat chakra.
Heart chakra;
Solar Plexus chakra.
Active energy.

WHY

When the focus is on a specific need to express the 'Self' in the most effective way without inviting conflict, this group comes into play. Passive energy softens the Solar Plexus energy and active energy stimulates the Throat.

Conversely, negative energy trapped in the Heart chakra can impede this free expression and we feel misunderstood or defensive when trying to explain ourselves.

We can actually feel our chest tighten in these circumstances.

A free flow of energy or a conscious awareness inviting positive chakra energy from the other two can help us to communicate more easily and clearly. It also prevents us from imposing our will/ego on events and others.

Group of three lower physical chakras.

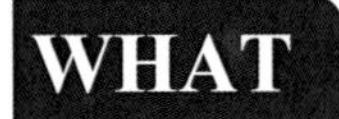

Solar Plexus chakra.
Sacral chakra.
Root chakra.

WHY

- *growth/development* from Sun of Solar Plexus above.
  (+ water from kidneys/large intestines)
- *Reproductivity* from **Sacral** chakra.
- *growing medium/nourishment* from Earth of **Root** chakra below.

This after all is the area where fertilization and development of the zygote (fertilized egg) into embryo occurs;

- Our promise of and for a future.
- The beginning of life.
- Fertility and growth.

HOW

Within this lowest chakra stage, the interior of the uterus is developing the placenta to feed the growing embryo from the mother's blood stream. All this initial growth and establishment of the new child and its environment is fittingly, in the **Root** chakra, the area of survival.

Internal growth and development.
Once this is established, the fœtus in the womb moves up to the mother's **Sacral** chakra as its gender is developing.

- As the uterus expands to accommodate the growing child, so it passes through all the mother's lower chakras.
- The stages of physical development correspond to the chakras baby passes through.
- Cerebral development is completed as the top of the uterus enters the mother's Solar Plexus chakra.
- The final stage in the ninth month: the child is tucked high up under the diaphragm and therefore enters the mother's Heart chakra just before birth.
- It is not for nothing that the breasts are either side of and encompass the Heart chakra.

External growth and development.
The Heart chakra is the centre of the spread of the thoracic spinal nerves to the periphery of the body. All these are intercostals (between ribs) so are effectively linked to the heart chakra. However, the lower 3 cross the solar plexus but the heart chakra influences and encompasses this outer area too. (*See Dermatomes* Chap**:** 10**, Fig:14.**)

These **heart** chakra intercostal nerve endings spread across the body, enveloping the torso from above the breasts to the pubic bone at the front and the small of the back, behind. This effectively covers the developing child in the expanding uterus. The **heart** chakra nerve endings also come down the inside of the arms to the palms, which are the physical contact when cradling a child.

> Thus the loving energy from this chakra is in contact with the new life growing within the mother's body throughout the whole pregnancy and during the feeding and care of the infant after birth.

The old saying that 'A happy mum is a happy baby,' is quite true. Understanding these biological and emotional energy connections is very important to both mother and child.

*****

Because the unborn babe shares the mother's energy system (s)he naturally responds to her conscious and subconscious feelings and emotions. And vice versa in the close interplay of energies after birth. This energy-sharing and close interplay in early life indicates why the mother-offspring bond is so strong and influential.

Where someone seems to 'pattern' aspects of the mother's issues/problems, especially daughters, this indicates that these have been absorbed by the offspring from strong patterns trapped in the mother's energy system. (Thus it is helpful to work on releasing personal and parental issues during pregnancy.)

Naturally, doubts and uncertainties come up related just to pregnancy. If they are accompanied by feelings of distress or fear about the pregnancy or anticipated pain and delivery, then clearing them from her energy system benefits mother, and unborn baby's energy system too. This is also the best time to clear any **Sacral** or **Pituitary** issues. (*See* pp120-125 & pp48-50)

Alleviating such anxieties and tension will improve the mum's energy and peace of mind. This is especially helpful in the last months. Labour and the delivery will benefit. Hormones will settle more readily when the lower chakras are harmonised.

Deeply suppressed fears and anxiety plus personal emotional issues prior to childbirth can readily undermine the mum's maternal feelings and expected joy in her new babe. Clearing them as soon as possible could avert and/or improve the distress of 'baby blues' and post-natal depression.

Between unsettled hormones and the huge change in a woman's life, she is particularly vulnerable to anxieties; even fear and distress about her own abilities to cope. These will readily block the flow of vitality in the centres and reduce both her mental and physical energy when she needs them most. Clearing the lower 3 chakras strengthens them for the active interplay needed for carrying the weight gained in pregnancy and the physical demands afterwards.

Immediate changes that both, especially first-time, parents have to contend with:-
- The constant needs/requirements/demands of a new baby.
- Disruption to/lack of sleep.
- Anxieties, real and perceived, about baby's health/thriving/feeding etc.
- Disruption to married life.
- Changes to relationship.
- New grandparents' requirements/issues.
- Physical image pressures.
- Peer pressure.(self/baby)

Expectation of the consequences is important. Discussing how these can be worked on together would relieve the emotional burden and help the relationship too. Even acknowledging anxieties and fears will make a difference. It could also bring up unrealized issues too. Getting rid of them quickly as they surface will prevent them from being buried again. (*See* ***Section 3***) The use of releasing techniques to relieve tension and anxiety beforehand will make it easier to make use of them afterwards as things come up. Any help to the emotional side of parenthood is worth the time.

In the case of deep fears and anxieties, frustration or anger, or even sorrow/deep despair associated with the pregnancy, looking at the **root** chakra sources and working to release as much as possible during the pregnancy will be very important as well as beneficial with regard to the shared energy system of mother and babe. After releasing techniques have relieved fear(s), any touch therapies, such as massage will be very therapeutic.

******

The phrase '*where (s)he's coming from*' is very true. Frequently it comes from one dominant energy centre. Most frequently the solar plexus, 'will/ego', and the 'sexual sacral' and the 'fearful root' centres are either dominant or inter-playing because all of these are strong energy centres. This can be either positive or negative in nature. Becoming conscious and aware of this dominance or interplay is a good way of realizing what is occurring, especially in a difficult or awkward situation. This makes it easier to appraise it less emotionally if negative responses are the result.

Dominance of one chakra can indicate unresolved issues relevant to the situation if different from the usual pattern of behaviour. If dominant as a general way of being, then the unresolved issues will be closely related to that energy centre. We can learn a lot about ourselves, and those closely inter-relating with/to us, from understanding where the dominant energy is emanating from, either habitually or under specific circumstances.

Equally, when one of the upper energy centres is dominant, that also is the focus of the exchange, for example if someone is being very vocal or over-demonstrative. If negative in nature, either it is in response to energy generated from another person or the situation and so related issues are indicated. There might be interplay from one of the lower active chakras which will also indicate unresolved issues if this is particularly noticeable. It is balance from the other passive chakras that modifies and enhances this use of energy.

Balancing certain chakra groups will change/enhance the dynamic of any situation. In a given situation, if it is possible, consciously focusing on one's own appropriate chakra group and calming the breathing can help achieve this. The response will be changed by this even if it is marginal and make the situation more manageable. Where you recognize repetitive issues occurring, making use of releasing techniques will enable better social interplay and greatly benefit all manner of relationships. When the related groups are in balance, relational interplay, therefore, is easier, comfortable and very rewarding.

Thus we are contributing unwittingly to the dynamic of any social/relational interplay. Part of where we ourselves '*are coming from*' sets the scene as much as the other(s) involved or the responses that result.

We can learn to harmonise our energy centre groups if we choose.

******

My Personal Notes

My Personal Notes

Section 3. Energy is The Key.

Energy is our life force, but negative energy dominates our lives and impairs our energy systems. In this section, therefore, we will take a closer look at the emotional energy we have covered in the preceding pages. Understanding why it is created, why it's there, what it's all for and how it all started will give you a much clearer idea of this vital part of our lives and health.

As you can see from the sources of negative energy we have looked at, the brain has a mass of negative energy and information influencing the thinking and reasoning it has to do. Naturally it will archive what thoughts and ideas it doesn't call upon on a day-to-day basis. But there will be a lot of negative energy caught up in the mass of electrical impulses flowing through the brain which is constantly filing away any related aspects in the association areas and memory. (*See* pp 42-3) It is all this that affects our general outlook and attitude, and of course our responses and reactions.

Fear, and pain its first cousin, underlie our emotions and readily lead to negative energy, so we will look first at them and why we have them.

Then we'll take a good look at the positive and negative why's and wherefore's of negative energy; its *function*, *nature* and *links*. Understanding these will be immensely helpful in gaining a better control of our lives and greater well-being. We all know *what* is negative. We need to understand *why*. Then we can do something constructive about it.

Knowing what it's really all about will have a positive effect, but knowing how to get rid of what is weighing us down will be much more effective. For this very purpose there is a chapter in this section on '*Visualisation Techniques*' to enable anyone to cut the ties to release themselves from the pain and negativity attached to memories and ideas and really restore warm invigorating energy.

This is essential to enable the free flow of life energy to be brought into play. Any work we do on our own negative issues will enhance any therapeutic treatment or healing practices, conventional or complementary, that we receive. It is the free flow of *positive* life energy throughout the body that is the ultimate aim of therapist and healer. The focus is the whole body and the work is to initiate the balance and harmony for the emotional and physical equilibrium so essential to healing. This can only come through understanding the way mind and body work together and the understanding and acknowledgement of as many aspects of that wholeness.

So that this book can be used as an on-going valuable reference, each aspect of energy here is dealt with as a complete unit so that certain significant points may be repeated in order to keep each part defined.

Just as we have explored the wholeness of the body through its internal connectedness, we will now explore the external inter-connectedness that is our relationship with the people and the world around us through that energy. This is a vital part of our lives.

Thus, understanding our energy in terms of how and why we 'relate' as we do is indispensable to our development and awareness of the quality of life we are experiencing.

This section therefore is to help:-
1) To realise fully the vibrational power of our personal energy. We are responsible for whatever that vibration has become. We are the creator and *we emit* it.
2) To recognize that responsibility, that what we initiate *will* set up the response or reaction that creates our experiences.

However, we need to be conscious that even without encountering people we vibrate with our environment: a room, a building, the ambient air outside creating a collective energy. We are truly connected and one with our environment and our world.

Becoming aware of this and consciously working to ensure that our energy vibration is as warm and vital as we can make it, is the purpose of this concluding section.

Chapter 16. Nature's Tools for Learning.

All living creatures were given an essential primæval tool to help the brain teach us to survive.

That tool was the emotion, *fear*.
It was 'task-specific', to *assess* and *learn* from every experience.
Every lesson was stored in the memory and each one increased the chances of that individual staying alive long enough to reproduce.

For such a fundamental and vital task, it had to be really effective, over-riding even. This basic protective emotion is totally instinctive and lies in the subconscious brain.

That primitive function of fear has not been diminished over time during our development into modern man from our ancestral *homo sapiens*. Our emotions are now as complex and sophisticated as our thinking abilities. However, fear is by its nature a negative energy and some very complex and negative thinking has developed with our brain! And from a tool for survival fear has now also become a two-edged sword: one side to use against others and the other, alas, against ourselves. Aren't we good at thinking negatively against ourselves? We believe something bad or negative about ourselves far more quickly than we do anything good!! - Don't we?

All first communication between living things is on the sub-conscious level and dependent on internal memory and linked external stimuli that jog our memory banks.

The subconscious sends out 'feelers' or vibrational signals for our initial contact with all other species. There is also a sub-conscious initial response: determined also by that original survival instinct. This is the essential *start* of our communication system. Sophistication of speech, thinking and man-made forms of communication have moved our consciousness away from this basic principle so its significance is much overlooked.

However, haven't we all said,
'My instincts told me…'
'I knew/felt instinctively…..!'
'I wish I'd followed my instincts!'
'I took/didn't take to her/him from the very first!'
'My (first) instincts are never wrong!'

Such familiar phrases. But how often do we over-rule them? We have more faith in our cerebral, conscious thoughts and powers of 'reason'.
However, thinking always comes *after* sub-conscious appraisal. It is so fast, we don't realise it.

Conscious communication, therefore, is secondary and is stimulated by further visual information and mental calculation. We base this on selected and appropriate memory; but the brain will also add to the pot any stored or buried associations so that we are well prepared for the event or situation. We tend to believe in it more readily because it's very rapid and more complicated; we've 'thought' it, so it must be ok.

But it is also subject to bias thanks to our complex emotions; conscious and subconscious of course. Any negative associations will be part of our interpretation of our experiences. And negativity usually distorts things.

The brain is like a sponge: it absorbs and remembers *everything,* for everything is potentially useful for survival. It has five senses to help accomplish this after all! Everything is carefully stored in our memory banks for possible future use for our protection.

Memory helps us survive. Fear is the tool for it because we remember what we fear most clearly. This is the primary biological function of knowledge as far as the brain is concerned, the assessment and interpretation of danger and survival.

Thinking and reasoning came much later and gradually both have become very sophisticated and complex thanks to man's social and technological development. But thinking and reasoning are incidental to the brain's original biological function which is naturally still there.

Still busy at protection and survival techniques, the brain tucks away *all* of what it learns for future contingencies and reference; but what disturbs us, what our 'conscious' upper brain doesn't like, or rejects as too unpleasant, *ie: is emotionally unacceptable*, it buries. In the sub-conscious, where fear has its origins.

How many negative emotions have their origin in fear?

Those phrases, *'Oh, I've dealt with that!' 'That's so long ago, it doesn't bother me!'* and similar quotes, make us believe that a problem, issue, fear, emotion has somehow vanished; we've 'thought' it away. No. We have suppressed it. It's now down in the archives. And the stronger the emotions and issues are, the less palatable or acceptable they are, the deeper we bury them. They will be part of our energy.

The human spirit does have amazing abilities to rise above them, for people are strengthened by adversity. We seem to learn best from hard knocks…back to that original need for fear to learn to survive by! We can rise above it with the conscious desire and effort to get on with things. But note the phrase 'rise above it'. *It's still there.*

But we mustn't over-look the fact that many of us keep the unpalatable, the fearful, etc just under the surface to look at now & then, or even as a 'companion', out of a need to punish ourselves. Or, it has to be said, to punish others with. Very often from a subconscious need or cause that *is* deeply buried. But as well as this agenda, our subconscious *is drawing our attention to it* as a reminder of what we are doing to ourselves. For if we use some issue against another person, *we will receive a negative result back* in some form or another. This is also part of a self-punishing cycle, which, again, needs to be recognized and acknowledged.

> But when the brain buries something, the body will reflect it, manifest it, suffer from it, because *the body and mind are one.* It has to come out somewhere, because it's there!

Any conscious or subconscious reminder that is remotely connected or related to what is buried will link up with it.

> Think of fear as a magnet that attracts memories to it for survival.

If a memory is related in any way to the fear impulse, it will become attached. Negative memory is second cousin to fear. Anger, resentment, hatred, frustration are heavy energy. Think of each one as a magnet too. Each attracts metaphorical filings, nuts, bolts, every scrap of the same nature. And since each piece in turn becomes 'magnetic', so more is attracted, ad infinitum, creating a veritable 'magnetic', ie: negative, field! And denser and heavier it gets too! Gravity being what it is, it descends to make us feel leaden in both spirits and body.

It is here, in the secret, hidden and largely dismissed area of the subconscious, that negative and positive energy is absorbed and transmitted. This is actually 'where we are coming from'. This determines not only our social inter-action but our *mental well-being and ultimately our health.*

> Whatever goes on in our mind goes on in our body.

But although nothing ever leaves the memory, it *is* possible to release memories from the dark/unpleasant emotions that go with them. Once that is accomplished, the mind has a better chance of dealing with issues and problems through positive conscious thought and action. This makes good use of the memories as signposts. Those things of the past do not then haunt us and tear at us destructively in our subconscious. Instead, they lie quietly doing no more harm until we need them as a tool for wisdom and knowledge *of ourselves, and what we are and can be capable of.*

Fear then is a useful tool once more, not a controlling factor in our lives and a stick to beat ourselves and others with along the way.

To ensure this, there is a simple and effective method that does *not* entail re-living those rather-be-forgotten experiences. Re-living them merely brings them up into the conscious brain which *still* doesn't like them; so it will bury them again as quickly as possible with emotions attached as before.

We can neutralize negativity by *positive thinking and outlook* readily enough *if we set our minds to it,* but this really is only a *surface remedy*. Remember, the brain is hanging on to *all* of it in case it comes in useful! Have pity on it and do less 'beating our brains out' with negative thoughts, ideas and emotions by learning how to let them go. If we can release these to give the brain a break, we will gain considerable peace of mind and our energy system will benefit enormously as well!

The releasing method is to cut the emotional ties. This comes at the end of this whole section in Chapter 21, when all the aspects have been covered. This is for 'clearing' away negative energy and changing it to positive physical and mental vitality.

******

Fear and pain work together for survival.

Both actually have positive attributes, but both lead readily to negative energy. We don't like feeling either of them, but if we can understand the positive side of them, they will become less of a monster we would rather avoid. We quickly learn the consequences of danger from fear, for personal safety. And we learn it often through the physical pain that results. This is to teach us to avoid the same situation and be aware of it and we do: eg: not to touch anything hot, otherwise we get burnt.

However, in animals, hunger or defence of the young makes them take risks. So we have this inbuilt too. Sophisticated man, who has mastered his environment, feels that he can take more sophisticated risks, but he has developed reasoning so that he can understand the consequences clearly too.

Situations of risk and knowing the likely consequences will involve anxiety, fear and mixed emotions. And yet we still take them! We like the buzz, for then we feel sharply aware, more alive and often empowered. We are challenging life. We need to.
Fool-hardiness is different; it is ego-driven. But this riskiness is attached to fear.

This is a positive aspect of fear which teaches us about ourselves in challenging situations while developing ourselves and our life-skills in the process.

The negative energy generated by the fear in these instances might make us feel drained or tired afterwards, but is balanced out quite soon by the positive consequences.

Fear is a boundary, but one that we need to assess. It is needed both to give us time to consider the consequences and a barrier we need as a challenge to break through. Fear therefore helps us to push against boundaries, especially those within ourselves. But it saves us from recklessness and teaches us discernment. Realisation that fear is a tool can do much to help us not to fear 'fear' itself.

When fear arises, we need to ask ourselves what it is trying to tell us.
And then follow through truthfully.

Hiding from it, ignoring it, trying to run from it allows it to become negative energy that invades the energy centres and system. We feel tired, out of sorts and confused. This is most unhelpful because it suppresses our ability to deal with what is happening.

Fearing fear itself, increases it - to our detriment. However, thinking of it as a tool for learning and understanding will put it to good use and have positive results which will counteract it.
Used properly, our survival as an individual is greatly enhanced.

To learn from it we need to ask ourselves *why* we feel the fear and anxiety and be truthful to ourselves about it. Is it based on a memory or association and creating the stressful situation? If it *is* attached to something, then that is what needs to be dealt with. This shows us why we have the fear and what we do to ourselves as a consequence. In clearing it, we free ourselves from the emotional pain and anxiety and clear the thinking so that the present situation can be tackled. If it is a present fear about doing something, then we need to assess the probability that it would be wiser not done, unless the consequences of doing it are something we can or wish to deal/cope with.

******

Example scenario:-
You have been asked to present something in front of colleagues/management etc (or it could be part of a job you want.)
Immediately there is apprehension:
- Fear of being humiliated/feeling stupid/can't control nerves/voice etc
- Anticipation of nausea/being sick/upset stomach; making a fool of oneself; being fired.

However, it is a challenge and the consequences will be positive - but the fear sends you around in a circle so that you can't think clearly. Apprehension, denial and even self-pity don't help. It's easy to feel trapped in them.

WHAT
Work out exactly *what* you fear and feel, and clear that.

WHY
Then look into your memory. Perhaps you were, or saw someone criticised/humiliated, even scared when either 'speaking up' (to parent, in class etc) or speaking publicly. Maybe other people have told you they were 'scared/terrified'; so you believe you will be too. If so, then clear these aspects as well.

Now you will discover:-
- What emotions a past memory can bring up.
- Why you were scared or reluctant to do something.
- How you can face and deal with a challenge you thought you didn't want/couldn't do.
- To avoid a situation inviting criticism by being prepared with what you are presenting or approaching a critical person in a different way.
- You can avoid setting up negative thinking in others.

In this way fear has been used properly and a person is in control of events and the self, without enduring an ordeal of nervous tension that sets up another memory for fear to hook on to.

HOW

By removing the bonds that tie us to doubt and fear, which the releasing techniques in tie-cutting* described in Chapter 21, allows you to do. Then, having cleared the emotional ties, the memory remains to remind us of the event. But next time it can be faced with just the right amount of current tension to make one work at it to make the presentation good. Memory is then a *reference*, not something to cut yourself on!

Through helping people with many aspects of fear, I often hear the phrase, '*I've lost my confidence'*. I have discovered that the reason many people put off or decide against doing something is because what they are really afraid of is that they might find out that they *can't* do it. ie: it will prove they are feeble/useless/too old/lacking in ability etc! Releasing the thought '*I'd hate to find out I can't/couldn't do it*'(* see above) enables people to make that step to discovering that, after all, they can.

Pain is also something we need to understand: one because we don't like it, and two, it usually makes us seek help for it. We seek healing as an end to pain, but knowing something about pain itself will help us to choose what to do about it.

Pain is also a tool for learning. It is not to 'teach us a lesson' in the punitive sense; (that's a negative!) it is the beginning of learning to find the cause and the cure. It is a *consequence*… of something else,…not a punishment.

Pain, therefore, should be the beginning of change.

Pain is the first signal that something is wrong and is to draw our attention to what needs *understanding*. Yet we can't wait to cover it up, ignore it and hope it will go away. (This goes for physical *and* emotional pain.)

While finding the organic cause of pain might be in the hands of others, managing pain and understanding our responses to it and dealing with it, is in *our* hands.

Pain is caused by pressure on a nerve or being passed on through the nerve network. It can be caused by muscular spasm, injury or disease *and* emotional tension: ie: any degree of physical and emotional trauma or negative thinking.

If proof is needed of the reality of heavy negative emotion being trapped in the body, the pain in tense muscles of, for example, the head, neck & shoulders, is exactly that. Pain and illness can and are exacerbated by very understandable negative emotions:-

- Anticipation/expectation of further pain.
- Belief that '*It'll never go away*'

• Negative thoughts: eg: *'I hate this', 'I'm stuck with this', 'It doesn't seem to be getting any better', 'It's spoiling/controlling my life', 'I can't get on with things'*, etc.
These will cause a lot of tension so that the muscles become stiff and unresponsive, making the situation worse. The body then moves more awkwardly causing further aches and pains. It's more likely then to strain or pull muscles, tendons or ligaments.

When the body is so muscularly unbalanced, a *physical-emotional* cycle is created.
The doubts and confusion will block the **Crown** chakra and the frustration/resentment/ bitterness will block the **Root** chakra. Thus their energy will be depleted making one feel even less well.

It is so easy to feel swamped by the pain and how rotten we feel. It can take over very quickly and fill the mind. But a concerted effort not to let it overcome one plus becoming *aware* of the muscular tension the body is under as a result can do much to start the process of helping ourselves turn the tables on the situation.

But we need know *why* we have pain. The illness, injury, etc, (ie: the physical *cause*) is a result of something. **Pain is a symptom**. There will always be an underlying reason from emotional issues from some source. Emotional tension will also intensify pain from an organic source. Interpreting the site of the pain can lead us to any emotional issues.

By looking at where the pain is and identifying what connection or connections it has, we can interpret it from our understanding of the body's anatomical and energy systems we've looked at, because the nerves and their pathways transmit energy. (Any work on the energy system therefore can and does relieve pain.)
By connecting the pain to a source of an emotional problem or issue, clearing that will also relieve the pressure in the area and surrounding tissues. Then relief and healing can begin to take place.

HOW

- Identify the energy centre/chakra area the pain is in.
- Look at sources of negative energy (*see* both organs & dermatomes) and identify.
- Ask: 'What is bothering me at the moment?'
  Has something been an issue for a long time?..Lying dormant? Keeps coming up? Keep remembering? A situation you dislike/fear?
- Which side of the body is it?
  - Right is the male principle.
    (look to **solar plexus/root** causes of negativity also)
  - Left is the female principle.
    (look to **brow/sacral** causes of negativity also)

The connections you make as you identify some source might even reveal something else you have forgotten about, something that is also connected by memory or association to what is currently causing you concern. The current issue or concern could be just lurking beneath the surface because we would rather not look at it. But distress, anxiety, annoyance, frustration, remorse, guilt or even fear, will show itself, even if it's in a headache or indigestion! Your body will tell you! If you really want to help yourself, deal with what comes to the surface by clearing it.

Emotional pain will often go to the site of an old injury and make it painful, or you will injure an old site, both of which means it is being *drawn to your attention* by your inner self and needs dealing with. Giving a few moments thought to what emotional situations or events happened then and currently will really pay dividends.

Once identified and acknowledged, issues and problems can be cleared. Sometimes a solution presents itself that wasn't there before. If not, cutting the emotional ties will prevent it from being buried again and causing further physical effects. It will be out of your system and the body's healing capabilities will have free rein.

We usually do learn the lessons from physical pain. However, we find it difficult to learn from emotional pain not to go through it again. That's because emotional pain gets buried because we don't like it. We cannot re-live physical pain, only remember we didn't like it much. But we *can* re-live emotional pain; so it is very powerful indeed. Why? Because it is and can be a destructive force which we need to learn about properly and control.

And the body *will* be physically affected by it in some way or other.

It is our reminder, our messenger. It tells us what is wrong. So we need to help the body all we can. And we can if we wish to. Understanding the origins of fear and pain and the complex emotions connected to them and how they relate to you and affect your body *can* help you to deal with them.

Releasing the negativity through the methods described in Chapter 21 really pays off. Once you have tried, it you'll realise pain can be managed. Also much can be done to relieve emotional tension through relaxation techniques and therapeutic treatments.

All this also applies to the fears, anxieties and uncertainties, even self-pity, that accompany being ill…from every degree from being unwell to any pain-free illness. The worries from '*What if…?*' questions are frequent unspoken fears that go through people's minds at such times. It is hard to make an effort to stand back from ourselves and look at what we are feeling and thinking at such times, but if we can, much can be done to help ourselves by changing our mental outlook through exploring those thoughts and feelings. .

Make a note of them and deal with them thoroughly. Releasing yourself from the weight of them in your energy means you will feel a lot less depleted and cope much better mentally. Then the body is better able to deal with the illness or injury. Every time you are miserable, your body's in a funk too.

******

Chapter 17. The Nature Of Negativity.

So what is it all for?

Well, we do actually need negativity.
Just as fear is essentially a tool, so is negativity.

Shadows or darkness make us aware of the quality and quantity of light.

We need the contrast to see that the light is there. We usually act upon the contrast: we switch on more light; light a candle; cover up warmly if it clouds over. And isn't there always a moment of disappointment as light diminishes? We always realise *what* has changed and it makes us *do* something about it.

Negativity always brings a measure of darkness to our day, our thoughts and our *perspective* on things.

Do we realise what has changed and act upon it as we would with physical darkness such as at dusk or night-time?

We wouldn't dream of stumbling about in the dark if we had a torch, candle or light switch to light things up. If we hadn't, we'd stop and let our eyes get accustomed to the dark before we moved about, wouldn't we?

Yet in the dimness, or darkness of negativity we are so absorbed by it that we don't think to light a light.

More often than not we stumble about and lose our way! We accept the 'darkness' without question! It's not so obvious as if a fuse has gone, there's a power-cut, night has fallen or even if it has gone cloudy. We'd react to those.

So in emotional darkness we need to ask ourselves '**why?**' What drew it? What is it in response to? Why do we feel negative or why are we in a negative situation? Then we'd be able to act on it to dispel that gloom or blackness that shadows the mind.

So it is a tool to draw our attention to things; to find out what we are doing and are allowing to happen to *ourselves*, or even to others. It is our tool of assessment; to make us take notice; consider our options; rethink our actions. Sometimes we have to bump into something to realise it's there. That teaches us to look where we are going and avoid it in future. So it is with the negativity. We need it to learn from, just as its 'first cousin' fear, was an original tool to learn from.

Negative situations are invariably our own creations. We either allow a response in ourselves, or actually invite negative energy and situations by sending out our own because subconsciously we need and want to learn something useful. We don't have a convenient alter ego chatting to us to tell us what's what. However, we do have our subconscious selves using our negativity and negative energy to prompt us. This is to get us to *take notice* of important lessons for our quality of life and development. Through real awareness and understanding of the *why* of what we are doing and what is happening, we are in charge of our lives.

If we view negativity in this way, we are less likely to be dragged down by it and get so bogged down that we don't really think to help ourselves. Then our conscious brain wouldn't go to all that trouble to hide the problem!

For once hidden, left to fester, given lots of negative attention to keep the pot of misery stirred or anger boiling etc, it becomes destructive stored negative energy. *It wants us to learn.* But if we don't, it increases like a nagging child to get our attention. Thus we compound it or ignore it until illness, injury or disease, which is really a great *big* shout, is the result.

We need to consider briefly these two aspects within the nature of negative energy.

Hot energy.
This invariably seeks to be externalized.
Anger, Rage, Resentment, Frustration - these will come out/boil over, somehow.
By its nature this energy will expand and spread negativity outwards to the whole area.

We know how hot we get when we are really angry; so we can see that this then spreads throughout the whole energy system. This will rapidly engage with the energy centre of the other person or people involved. Naturally, this will create a reaction which then bounces back to us. Diffusing this situation is therefore important to both parties, especially since we can't fully realize what issues it can affect in the other person.

Cold energy.
This is very internal and personal.
Sorrow, Grief, Hatred, Cold spite - these will be suppressed and stay inside us.
By its nature this energy will consolidate.
This will be like carrying a stone inside and intensify any negative energy internally.

This is very damaging to the carrier. It will form a cold vibration. The response of either rejection, being shunned, disliked, even hated will also rebound on the carrier.

However negative thoughts and fears are different. Thoughts are always in the cerebrum. Negative ones can be neutralised by a positive outlook if you make the effort not to let them linger. Reversing a negative statement or thought to a positive one as soon as possible does wonders. (Try it. You'll actually discover your own negativity.)

However, it is letting them fester, from dwelling on them to convince oneself that they are true and meaningful, (and we do rummage through them like a rack of sale goods, don't we?) that they can *become* a fear and a 'magnetic hook' for similar negative associations.

But before we can deal with this dark energy we need to look at it and see how it works.

By looking at the principles of positive and negative energy, and getting to know how it comes into being, we will have a better idea of what we are up against. Understanding its nature and how it becomes destructive will help in clarifying problems or issues and help initiate a solution. The next chapters are to help you do that.

It is by understanding and accepting our issues, problems and negativities and then determining ways to deal with them, that is really to take responsibility for our lives. We each of us determine the quality of the way we live anyway. In which case, we can improve it once we know how and why. Then we can strengthen our emotional inner core and help our physical core to work at its best. This really helps us to stand on our own two feet.

******

My Personal Notes

Chapter 18. Principles of Positive and Negative Energy.

Having explored the sources of internal and external energy through the relevant anatomy, it would be helpful now to understand the nature of energy, ie: the way energy behaves and inter-acts and is generated. But most importantly, how and *why.*

The nature of energy is such that should it impact on a recognised source/conductor of the *same* energy, it will then *re*-generate from it and return to source creating a link along which the energy can travel back and forth. (eg: Direct current in electricity)

The only way to stop the energy from rebounding/regenerating is to change the substance of the *receptor* and therefore the response will be changed/deflected, (the principle of Alternating Current in electricity - which, incidentally, makes it more controllable!).

It is exactly so with all living species.

All *generated* energy initiates a response:

eg: a beam of light striking a surface illuminates and spreads;
a tennis ball hitting an obstacle bounces using the energy transmitted by its impact.

The nature of the energy remains unchanged but the response is determined by what it encounters. So energy will *re*generate from any impact, using the energy generated by the impact.

Negative energy is a generated energy.

Positive energy just '*is*'.
It is there because all living matter is positive energy. However, it has a vibration or pulse which will respond:-

- when encountering and/or recognising a similar positive vibration,
- to the energy from a negative vibration.

In all the cellular activity of the body, chemical bonding of particles occurs through recognition, ie: their *proper orientation.* To form these bonds *takes* energy. The breaking of them, *creates* energy. This is a natural continuing process in all living cells. This metabolic process is essential to give our bodies the energy constantly to replenish itself and be a living organism.

In the same way, negative energy, in **forming** a bond with negative energy, **uses** energy.
The **breaking** of these bonds, **creates** energy.
The creation of this energy is in the inter-action of positive and negative energy.

This is what we need to bring about: creating energy by breaking the bonding of negative energy to itself and particularly the initial 'magnet' of the under-lying issue or problem.

The energy we *use* for this process is mental energy, both conscious and subconcious.

Left alone,

- negative energy increases in density through bond-forming.
- uses up the positive energy.
- inhibits creation of energy by no bond-breaking.
- increases inertia in energy centre.
- less movement = more inertia = increased inhibition of bond-breaking.
- has potential for expansion into surrounding areas.
- continually taking energy.
- less energy available = increased density of negative energy.

1) In order to effect change, there needs to be a collision of particles to create fresh energy.
2) By the release of any negative energy, change can occur.
3) Healing and therapeutic methods can then send positive vibrations into the area to act as that 'excitability' needed to stimulate the collision factor for bond-breaking to occur.
4) This will create positive energy to displace the inertia of the negative energy.
5) This surge of energy initiates the healing process.
6) It can be clearly seen that release and change of negative energy needs to be thorough so that the energy centre is cleared and able to function correctly for the body's benefit.
7) The conscious awareness of this process and the application of release and healing/therapy will ensure that there is a constant inter-reaction between negative and positive energy to boost the energy centres and maintain homeostasis.

The quality of relationships of all kinds, from personal, business or inter-social activity of all kinds will be determined by the energy that is *generated* by us. We need awareness of what we generate and why, so that we grow in understanding of the responses that make up our communication with others.

*****

Serious issues from darker emotions accompanying sexual negativity causing a shutting down of social response (introversion/aversion/frigidity etc) as a protective measure, can be better understood through knowledge of the **sacral** and **root** areas and the actual nature of negative energy. If deeply trapped, causing aggressive and/or dangerous and even obsessive issues*, they can be seen to be rooted in the survival instinct and linked to the limbic system. (*See* Chap: 3) (*This area is more complex than this book covers.)

Chapter 19. The Negative Response Cycle.

Animals act on the instinctive survival level. They all know unerringly what the response should be and act accordingly, because they mostly have *'one initiation, one response'* in place at a time. This in animals is in turn, stored as a *positive* use of negative energy.(a natural *resource*) Their memory store is all for *learning to survive.* Fear in the given moment stimulates the correct response as a protective device. So it was with primæval man. It is *the* basic emotional response that is designed specifically to ensure survival through learning about threats and danger.

However, Man developed further through his growing sophistication of thought and communication.

> The Human Being has the added factor of higher consciousness. Our complex thinking means we have *imagination* and this enlarges and classifies all the different things that our brains experience as a variety of things to fear.

Sadly, humans readily:-

- live in fear,
- re-live fear,
- dwell on fears,
- perceive/anticipate fears un-necessarily.

When we torment ourselves with our complex memories and associations, it ceases to be a tool for learning.

The result is an intricate system of negative links and consequences.
The majority of our *connections* and *responses* are on the sub-conscious level.

Thanks to the sophisticated human cerebral development that buries what we don't like in our 'archives', all the uncomfortable or horrible things dismissed from our minds sit deeply in the subconscious. With all the other memories they *send out unconscious pulses which encounter others that they then respond to.*

Humans have become destructive with negative energy by allying it to *the intellect.*
We compound it cerebrally through our thinking and use it sub-consciously *or* consciously, to hurt ourselves and others.

This effectively *disempowers* us.

Negative thinking is to give away your power.

Encouraging negative thinking from others or taking their negativity personally is to disempower yourself also, because it saps your energy or fuels more negativity within you. This goes for negative *attitude* and *actions* as well. People use this negative 'bat and ball' both consciously and subconsciously to disempower others or one another. They feel empowered by it as it brings up the adrenalin. However, they are actually giving away their own energy - adrenalin uses energy after all, and they will feel either flat or drained afterwards as the adrenalin subsides. This easily clouds the judgment and negative thinking usually follows: eg: resentment, feeling ill-used, fault-finding etc. This sets up a damaging negative cycle that re-bounds on the individual because they don't or won't let it go. Negative responses will be drawn to them as a result.

> This invariably sets up a fresh need for the adrenalin to give the person their sense of power, but that is all it is: the *feeling* of power, not power itself because they are giving it away and depleting themselves.

With the build-up of negativity replacing their positive energy, their chakras and system become blocked, leading to the physical and emotional problems we've already looked at. To re-energise themselves a cycle of need for the artificial stimulation from this negative 'bat and ball' establishes a pattern of behaviour in relationships and is both self-punishing and punishing to others. Fuelled by the negativity from other people's opinions and responses, the self-punishment is increased further. But the person is under the illusion of empowerment.

It is by the 'victim' allowing, in other words sub-consciously, or consciously agreeing to their use of aggressive power, that this person's negative adrenalin can be re-charged. This is always in the hands of the recipient. You'll receive it if you let it. Releasing your reasons *why* you accept or agree, sets you free.

Adrenalin used negatively stimulates testosterone because the survival impulse feels threatened. No-one is happy with the resulting negative outlook and aggressive attitude and behaviour. The Limbic brain is in charge. (*See* pp35-37)

This is different from 'having a row to clear the air'; that is a short-lived situation and a release of feelings and negative thoughts.

****

Because the heaviest negative energy gravitates down to the lower chakras and adrenalin is related to the **root** chakra it is helpful to note their physical relationship.

The 3 lower physical, active chakras are *closer together*:
3rd Solar Plexus......Intellect, will, ego...but also enlightenment.
2nd Sacral.............Sexual energy (physical activity/sensuality/reproductivity)
1st Root...............Survival/defence/earth connection.

Notice the *ascending* order towards the aspirational/spiritual passive upper chakras.

Our productive development towards enlightenment and higher knowledge needs to rise above the basic instincts and their energy in order for us to savour our potential and develop as mature and fulfilled human beings.

Blocked with **negative** energy, these lower chakras are damaging, even destructive;

- To the self......inhibits body's natural healing/energising processes.
- To others......attaches/stimulates/intensifies their negative energy.

Freely energised and **flowing** with **positive** energy, these lower chakras are productive and strengthening. The results are on-going and lead to more positive responses

- For health and well-being.
- To give impetus, ie: *active energy*, to the passive upper spiritual chakras.

This vitalized energy gives impetus to the conscious awareness to follow actively the higher thought and guidance of the upper aspirational/spiritual chakras.

This Active Positive energy also strengthens the Will and the Ego to give better control of our lives. Then we can develop as individuals and find improvement in our relationships.

An ego cleared of negative issues feels no need to prove itself.
'I want..' is from the Will.

A subconscious attitude of **'see me'**, means you feel you have to prove yourself. This is an act of will, ie: 'I want you to/you *will* like/approve of me'. People then *react* to you, which invites judgments and assumptions. Subconsciously emitting an **'I am me'** vibration, means .people will *respond* to you because you are subconsciously and even consciously comfortable to them.

Situations and relationships will develop smoothly and naturally in response to your inner security in being yourself.

******

My Personal Notes

Chapter 20. Understanding Negative Links.

The aspect of concern is that of Negative *links being created:-*

> **Negative energy, 'meeting' a negative response, *returns* and creates a link along which all further negative energy from both internal and external sources can, and does, travel.**

All sources of *internal* negativity, therefore, are a magnet to negativity.
If we wish to understand and change, then we need to ask ourselves 'why' of anything that resonates with us.

Guilt.
The guilt explored here is not that from actual wrong-doing or a conscious act(s) against someone/others, crime etc. That is being guilty of something. That is between the individual and his/her conscience. The fundamental knowledge of knowing right from wrong is the truth within that we cannot deny and which won't go away.

> This is not about judgment; it's about awareness and acknowledgement.

Guilt. no 1) Internal.
The guilt we put ourselves on the emotional rack about.

The Sense of Guilt/feeling guilty about eg: tactlessness, unintentional hurts, feeling you have let someone/people down, or haven't done enough/failed something/disappointed someone/oneself etc.

There are many small things we feel guilty about.

That's fine…it teaches us to be more careful and aware.

It's when we torment ourselves and turn a molehill into a mountain with dread and self-criticism that it becomes destructive instead of *a tool for learning caution and care.*

Guilt readily sets up a magnet, linking it to every little 'guilt' you feel. A detrimental negative cycle is the result.

Guilt. No 2) External.
This is the guilt we are *made to feel* by someone who is manipulating our vulnerable/caring/easily self-punishing self.
This sets up negative links quite quickly in relationships of all kinds.
You are allowing someone power over you to empower themselves.

These create negative energy against the Self.

- It attacks our self-concept and undermines our belief in ourselves.
- We want/need to sub-consciously punish ourselves.
- Belief that you deserve punishment/are bad/worthless.
- The martyrdom/self- crucifying syndrome.

If any of this is part of your life or experience you need to ask yourself *why* this is happening and, if you realise it is not what you want or choose, help yourself to release yourself from it.

Manipulation is a form of '**Agenda**' that we will be looking at next.

• If change is really wanted, there will be underlying issues for both parties that need to be addressed honestly.

• Sometimes both parties have a sub-conscious pact for this set-up that satisfies another agenda.

• This may be another parent-child need/habit from previous experiences/childhood.

Only the individual can choose to accept or change things.

Having Agendas.

Many people with personal issues stemming from negative situations, ideas, thoughts or perceptions carry 'agendas' into relationships either in the home or work-place. These become 'baggage' to all parties concerned and can vary from mild irritants to destructive habits.

Agendas are really about power and power-games. They achieve only negative effects. Life, and ultimately one's health, is not enhanced by this because it rebounds on us either by feeding our ego or poor self-concept. This then is really a *self*-defeating exercise; people with agendas have subconscious and conscious expectations/demands creating mental and physical tension and stress from the energy being exchanged between those involved. This can attract unpleasant even destructive attention to us.

It would be helpful now to look at these aspects which could be part of your own life or that of a client. Understanding these factors will assist in dealing with them.

Agendas are requirements *by* people *of* other people.

Emotional requirements are specific to relationships.

- Other people's 'requirement(s)' of you.
- Or your 'requirement(s)' of others.

I want - proof of your love, or remorse, your attention, recognition, sympathy etc.

Love/affection with '*requirements*' always creates a negative link between people.

'Requirements' are intrinsically negative as they involve *'I want'/expect* in some form.

- Subconscious.

  This is usually from personal insecurities, low self-concept, loneliness etc
  This induces guilt, anxiety, fear of failure etc in the other person(s) too.
- Conscious…ie: emotional blackmail.

  Requiring pity/sympathy/attention or the 'Ah! Poor me!' syndrome.

All these are very 'bat and ball' situations and lead to resentment, frustration from the pressure to fulfill these 'needs' and jealousy etc as well. This becomes an under-current to relationships and is often unquestioned and accepted. Either people become resigned or it is such a familiar habit it goes largely un-noticed.

This is a very negative cycle. It wears away at relationships.

Children often behave deliberately badly to test the strength of the parent/sibling's love/affection. *'If they still love me even though I'm naughty/bad/horrid etc, then I know they love me'* is a very common ploy for a child who is either insecure or is/feels ignored, and seeks any kind of attention. (Or are particularly egocentric and constantly desiring/demanding attention.) This latches onto the negative 'hook' of either guilt feelings or despair/frustration/anger in the other person at their sense of lack of control.

Unfortunately, many adults have kept up this pattern of thinking/behaving, though some transfer 'bad' behaviour into demanding/expecting/needing proofs in adult forms of expression or activity.

There are two-rôle relationships (eg: marriage/living together) that are founded upon a '*parent-child*' not '*adult to adult*' situation. This can stem from a sub-conscious need for the familiar pattern of a childhood relationship to continue. This could be the sub-conscious or even conscious choice in either one or both parties for either rôle.

Social conditioning also plays its part in this becoming established and an agenda for control/being controlled is set up as one 'spouse' automatically (often subconsciously) assumes the rôle of parent. The '*parent-child*' situation can lead to conflict here because it is not natural in an adult. S/he naturally assumes that s/he is 'grown up' and expects to be treated as such. This leads to a subconscious retaliation that shows in bickering and fault-finding etc. This, added to the underlying rôle situation, will lead to a negative cycle that is often quite damaging. It needs to be recognised.

Just as the fear of not being loved/liked creates agendas, pain and illness can cause them also. These can play their part in the '*parent-child*' rôle situation too.

It is important for anyone who wishes to follow the healing way of life, be it to help yourself or as a practitioner, to realise these agendas. Not all people wish to be healed. This needs to be understood and accepted until *the person him/herself chooses to make the change.*

Holding on to pain/illness - aspects of the Will - both adults and children.

1) Guilt/self punishment; conscious & subconscious - the Will against the self.

These all block the **Throat** and **Heart** chakras and slow the energy system as well.

- I deserve this/I am unworthy.
- People will think I'm faking if I get better quickly.
- It ought to/I expect it to hurt/make me feel bad.

- It was my own fault; I'm stupid so I need to feel pain/bad.
- We are here to suffer; other people suffer, so should I.

2) Negative Will/control/illusion of empowerment/Parent-child need.
These will all block the **Solar Plexus** chakra and those with the element of power will affect the **Root** chakra too. Anything against the self, blocks the **Heart** chakra.

- I like being/want to be dependent on her/him/people.
- I am a victim/I want to be/am going to be a victim.
- Victims get noticed/attention/sympathy/help.
- Once it stops I won't get noticed/any attention/help/sympathy.
- I need/it gives me, something to talk about.
- My pain's worse than his/hers/theirs.
- When people help me/sympathize, I am less frightened/alone/neglected.
- I can get her/him/people to do what I want/notice me/give me time/attention.
- It gives me power over her/him/people.
- I like/want her/him/people doing things for me.
- She/he/people ought to feel for me /my suffering.
- If I don't tell them, how will they know I'm a sufferer/ill?
- Life will change if the pain goes/I get better.
- I'm afraid of change/having to do more/cope with life/take responsibility.
- I can get out of things I don't like/want to do.

What also blocks the **Heart** chakra is holding on to grievances, real and perceived, ie: 'feeling hard done by' or deep resentments. (eg: emotional pain at break-ups, divorce etc.) Emotional separation, locking the feelings inside oneself especially with no company other than grievances is very damaging. These need to be let go.

Grief.
Through helping people come to terms with grieving in all forms of loss, I have learned that there are many aspects to it. However, grief at someone's death is the most sensitive subject. I feel that it is important enough to explore, especially for those who wish to understand it and those who truly wish to replace it with lovingness and relieve their hearts and minds of the burden of the pain of loss and the bitterness of remorse.

> This is *not* to trespass on the deep suffering of those whose loved ones die violently or in suffering. Releasing strategies may help to deal with it even in the early days or once the most harrowing thoughts fade so that life can be lived more easily in time.

In countries where there is uninhibited, loud and public displays of grief, such as ululation and keening, this vocal and physical 'expressing' acts as a great release. In the West death to us is desolation, and grief private and painful; to some it spoils their lives. We cry but keep it mostly locked inside us. People are embarrassed or non-plussed by other people's grief. Holding on to grief is very easily done and is invariably expected.

This and societies' judgments and expectations lead to agendas with grief. The most obvious is that of self-punishment from remorse which is a form of 'agenda against the self'. And remorse itself comes from quite complex issues.
The reasons for feeling the remorse need to be considered.
Are we feeling 'guilty' about something?

- Not making up in a row/burying the hatchet/being mean over something etc.
- Not showing/expressing enough love/caring/affection/visiting/doing enough?

But there are other agendas too.

- I want to hold on to them.(the person they have lost)
- If I don't think about grieving for them, I'll lose them completely/forget them.
- I should have been the one to die.
- Why did they leave me? It's not fair!
- If I don't show I'm grieving, people will think I'm heartless.
- I've got to keep it up to prove I loved/miss them, - to myself/to others.
- I must hide my feelings because other people don't want to know/be reminded.

These and thoughts like them put us under enormous pressure. They only deplete our energy. We forget, or think it wrong, that because we are left alive, that we should and can honour that and live happily and well. Releasing these gives us a chance to do that.

The sticks of remorse, anger, guilt and anxiety that we beat ourselves with are hard and often brutal. They just add to the pain of loss and compound the negativity, so that we feel crushed and washed out. As if the loss isn't enough. A loved one would not wish to leave a legacy like that for you. They would far rather we rejoiced in their life and having our life left to live and able therefore to hold the memory of them as a sweet and loving part of it. Remembering their life rather than their death, or even the one day they died, honours their memory and their life, as well as the life *you* have before you.

Release from Agendas: ...This will enrich one's life and relationships.

- *Realising* and *acknowledging* any agendas is the first step.
- *For the individual wishing to change things*, be free from the emotional bondage of pain and ill health that they have invited; releasing the fear of change/rejection/loneliness/pain/having no significance or value/desire for power/control etc.
- *For those under the control/manipulation of someone*, releasing one's own sense of guilt//pity/frustration/anger/need to be manipulated/poor self-concept that allows this.

Freely loving creates positive energy

- Internally.

'Being loving' neither requires, nor has expectations.
In this way negative links are not set up.

- Externally.

The change in what subtly emanates from *you* will effect change in others. because *you* will *initiate* a different *response.* The change will be subtle, but there will be change for the better.

Most people think of love in terms of emotion. Love isn't an emotion, it is just lovingness itself beaming from us and not involved with the will or ego.

Emotions are from the sensations and feelings we have regarding love or our idea of love, from tenderness right through to intense passion, or the emoting in hero/celebrity-worship. Emotion creates a vibration that influences the way the love is 'sent out'. Thus it is the *accompanying emotion* we need to identify and particularly what the result is for ourselves and others. What do we invite to ourselves from these emotions?

What requirements do we have from these emotions?

Emotions can and do cloud our judgment; so we need to ask ourselves whether we are viewing something difficult or perplexing from a purely emotional viewpoint. If you are, then, explore what you are *feeling* about it: have you felt like this before about something similar?. By thinking about 'why' you step back from the emotion. You are no longer 'in' it. Thus we are less likely to run headlong at the problem and set up a bad reaction, worry ourselves into a state about it or bury it for it to re-surface later. It could be hooked onto a buried one from previous times so this could help you unravel a pattern that takes you back to the original one that set it up. It's worth exploring.

We can easily set up an agenda that will rebound on us from not dealing promptly with emotional situations. Far better to choose to change things round to a positive outlook and 'letting it go', or even releasing all of it through visualisations etc.

There is also the requirement from the Will. With the best of intentions people, 'want' or 'think' that someone should respond in a certain way to their idea/requirement of what they should do or think. It can come from caring too much or a need/desire for power of some kind. A will-requirement, however, will rarely receive the response expected, it will only encounter the other person's will. Disappointment, resentment, frustration etc will be the inevitable result. Allowing someone free choice is to be loving to them. It is often the hardest thing to do. This enables lovingness to grow. Both parties have the chance to grow and develop. Releasing the need to 'bend someone to our will' saves a lot of wasted energy too!

The requirements and/or expectations people have of those they love, are close to, or are simply in their life usually dominate any relationship. Assessing whether we have these or what they are can reveal any issues that we have. Resolving them enables us to '*be loving*' and the response from others will change for the better because subconsciously - and sometimes consciously, they feel freer. This enables *their* love to flow freely too. Everyone benefits.

Therefore, in order to resolve the negativity buried in the sub-conscious that acts as a magnet and sets up this reciprocity, we need to deal with the sub-conscious 'problem' or issue and change the vibration ourselves with conscious awareness and visualisation strategies.

Cutting the negative links lets us do this. (described fully later in Chap: 21) It is a most effective way of releasing these emotional ties *without* re-entering or re-living the emotions and perceived hurts. Agendas can then be dropped. And agendas will always deplete the energy system and in turn one's health; so it's worth being rid of them.

Pity.
Pity takes two forms, to pity someone or to pity the self. We need to ask ourselves what pity means to us and what we do with it.

Feeling sorrow for the plight of someone needs to be compassionate. This is the true essence of what we call pity. Compassion is a loving caring which is generated from the inner being or heart as a healing vibration towards that person to support their endeavours. Compassion strengthens.

Pity is to think or imply that the other person lacks capability of self. This pity is a different matter. This is what people mean when they say 'I don't want your pity'. Everyone has hidden strengths and courage for adversity. Mostly this is kept private. To pity then is to negate that ability within the person, or any other capabilities they are making use of. It is actually therefore a judgment of their perceived lack. Thus pity weakens. Far better to send a silent conscious beam of encouragement as a strengthener to help them and believe in their strengths.

It is the same for self-pity.
We are judging ourselves as incapable of self-help from those same strengths of character, inner strength, courage, or any other abilities that we have as our tools for living. We are negating ourselves. We weaken ourselves. We need to ask ourselves why? Is it perceived as 'expected' thinking? Or perhaps we have an agenda? Do we want to weaken ourselves and invite more sympathy from others? Isn't it better to have compassion for ourselves in adversity or times of anything stressful? Mentally tallying up our own resources and sending ourselves a loving feeling of encouragement to deal with things is to strengthen the self from within. We can all do this.

We need to realize that self-doubt is not innate. We acquire it. Then we nurse it, feed it and give it full credibility! We do this with our will and ego. Emotions are very strong and negative ones have great power over us and consequently others.
We need to continue believing inside ourselves that we are not weak.

Acceptance.
We have become accustomed to accepting the 'that'll do' thinking of illness unless, happily, a specific cause and cure fit neatly together. We treat the symptoms or cover them up. Consideration and awareness of the whole picture of what ails us and really getting to the cause seems to be quite secondary. The body then has to struggle to function well in order to regain homeostasis.
The result is that the body is often under par and remains susceptible to further problems and ill-health. Why do we accept this?

There are several mind-sets about being unwell that seem quite valid to the individual and influence their approach to self-help/treatment/healing:-

- 'I haven't got the time.'
- 'It doesn't matter.'
- 'It'll go away with painkillers/time etc.'
- 'I can manage.'
- 'Suffering is noble/ennobling
- We are here to suffer/supposed to suffer.'
- 'It's what life's about.'

These have to be accepted as a person's choice. However this just indicates low self-concept and Will against the self. It is a shame that it prevents them dealing positively with what is under-mining their health. It is to be hoped that the change in today's thinking, that of seeking for and needing different answers to healing, better health and well-being, will encourage them to think differently about it.

I hope too that any reader who thinks 'that'll do', will have gained sufficient insight into concepts and issues from this book that they might do something to change that!

Acceptance is also in how much negative thinking and responses we readily allow to become part of day to day living. We don't realise it. It slips into the subconscious very quickly. However, it is quite easy to find out just how much by making a note of any negative thoughts or responses in the course of one day. It will probably surprise you. In the course of a week, you would get quite a clear picture of what you both *accept* and *don't question* regarding the quality of your life. Bringing it into your conscious awareness will begin the process of developing your life and looking to your well-being. Anything negative that is being repeated is begging for your attention!

> Once any negativity is identified, 'out in the open' as it were, its power decreases because it gives you the chance to be free of it.

Man is a complicated and complex creature; so pain, illness, suffering and healing are very complex issues that are bound up in many other issues. Healing can only begin to take place if this is understood and accepted as a whole set-up…and therefore *holistic*…that needs to be addressed by conscious awareness and willingness for change to true positive energy. This can only be decided upon by individuals themselves *for* themselves and as a consequence, for others. In this we *do* have free will.

This is as important for anyone concerned with *any* aspects of healing and care as it is for each individual. The condition of your health and your emotional perspective on life affect all that you do, how you relate to and work with others after all. It is an important consideration when assessing the quality of one's life in both personal and public spheres.

> When we can improve it ourselves, we empower ourselves in the best possible way.

The strength of emotion is known to us all; yet we rarely think of it as part of our health and condition. Even the word ‘stress’, which has become a modern buzz word, lacks real definition. Understanding and dealing with emotion and the body as a *whole unit* will bring a more enlightened view to health, and the healing we all need.

******

Chapter 21. Releasing Techniques. (Tie-cutting)

Now we will look at how to deal with and *change* negative energy.

WHY

- Negative energy makes *you* give *it* mastery over *you.*
- Negative issues in the sub-conscious means that the psyche controls *you.*
- *You* need to be the driver of your own car.
- To raise your own self concept by getting rid of negative concepts *against yourself.*
- Positive energy enables you to meet challenges with anticipation and overcome obstacles more easily.
- Positive energy is the enabler for all things good for the self.
- Subconscious positive energy means a positive attitude and vibration without having to use conscious effort. It then comes naturally.

Trapped negative energy needs to be shifted. We need to understand its pulling-power.

Effective releasing strategies:- Useful for,
- Discovering links.
- Breaking links.

They take moments to do, but one needs to be *willing, persistent* and *thorough.*
This is in order to cut the links along which emotional pain, anxiety, guilt, fear, etc travel from:-
- People.
- Events.
- Ideas.
- Habits.
- Anything that influences/controls your thinking.

It releases you from the negative link between you. It takes it *out of your energy.*

- It does *not* cut one off from a person you love or like.
- It enables you to *freely* love/like the person you are linked negatively to.
- It releases one's inner light towards the person you are linked negatively to.
- The link is cut within *you.*
- It can become **re**-attached if *you permit it through habit* or haven't been thorough and released the need for the habit. (*See* pp228-9.)

Cutting negative energy links creates *neutrality*; ie: release from anger, hatred, fear, from a person or people you dislike etc so that their negativity towards you is neutralized. Once in 'neutral' gear, (as in driving a car) you can chose to remain where you are or move forward in the relationship or situation. This gives *you* the choice.

Choice means that you can be in charge of what your life is about. The issues you clear are no longer in charge of *you*. Especially those against yourself that undermine you.

However, many people feel that they 'don't want to go there', or 'I don't want to think about it.' The important aspect of these releasing techniques is that you *don't* think about it. It's to do with visualization: ie: *seeing and looking at what the issue has created in your energy system.*

This does not mean that you 'see' the unpleasant event or person involved. It does not mean you dwell on the stressful or upsetting things which you are at pains to push aside or hide away. These will keep popping up into your thoughts anyway. Once they do come into your mind, however briefly, that will be all that is needed. Then using a releasing technique before you have time to dwell there will remove that emotional pain.

It's all about being willing not to tolerate the distress, hurt, anxiety etc, etc. And not go on being 'bullied' by those stresses and distresses. Nor waiting until you are feeling desperate, before you decide to deal with them. Pushing them aside, burying them will not make them go away, or give you time to 'pull yourself together', or 'get over it', or 'when I'm feeling better'. This is really only putting things off in the hopes it will all go away. It won't unless you work on them to give them up and free yourself from them.

Finding the courage not to accept or tolerate the negative things in life is far better.

WHAT

We can alter the subconscious negative vibration we impose internally on ourselves and what we emit or send out to others, through cutting the *emotional* links with memories. The memories remain; we need them. But the pain and fear etc that we experience from them is removed and with it the detriment to both mind and body.

We can do this through releasing them by cutting the ties described later.

This method is simple and does *not* involve re-living the emotion or trauma. That will only make the conscious mind bury it again as quickly as possible!

You need three things. **Willingness** above all, **Perseverance** and **Thoroughness.**
And the odd half an hour whenever you can spare it!

If we are willing enough, we can do a lot for ourselves and, as a *result* of what we *do* release for ourselves, other people in our lives too.

No one can change their nature. But we can make the best of our natures. We can develop as human individuals by conscious awareness of the human condition and by *changes in our own behaviour, outlook and attitude* and ultimately our personal value system. All these can be changed if we wish it.

This will initiate changes in *responses* from others; so situations will change around us.

If we can change our *subconscious* feelers or vibrations from negative to positive, in other words alter the *initial communication response* that is our first point of contact, the response will be instinctive because it is on the sub-conscious level. This will mean a change for the better in the behaviour and attitude of others toward you, but also, *you* will not have the link inside that will respond to *their* negativity if they hang on to it! And sometimes they do! It has become a habit with them. But look out for re-attachments! You might have the habit of responding too. The answer is to clear the attachment to thinking you deserve it.

Once our sub-conscious vibrations are clear, life changes. This helps our development. We also fear change less. Life in general gets a lot cheerier. By carrying a lot less angst, all aspects of one's life, especially one's health, improves. And good health always creates a positive subconscious vibration. When your inner vibration is more positive, others will respond more positively and so this is as much to do with clearing away *everyday* negative thoughts and ideas which make you feel low, tired, bored, fed-up, anxious, irritable or miserable.

*****

HOW

Now the nitty-gritty of these Releasing Techniques.

The great thing about this method is that *you* are in charge.

- Only you can decide to work on issues this way.
- Only you can do the visualisations and clear them.
- **Only *you* need to know what they are.**
- It's up to you how well you do it, no-one is going to tell you off or interfere if you aren't thorough. The results will be according to the effort though!
- You do *not* have to re-live the issues.
- You do not have to face or confront them.
- You are getting rid of the emotional links that you hurt yourself (and often others) on.

The whole business of link clearing is in picking up thoughts and visualization; seeing sentences or mental pictures. But **NOT** seeing damaging events or traumas.

<u>It is important to realise that you do not explore or re-live what troubles you.</u>

It is very important also *not* to ***think*** about the issue while you are clearing it; just concentrate on the clearing job; use your brainwork only for that: *looking* is the object.

There are several ways of tackling these negative thoughts, issues and problems which I have found effective for both myself and those I have helped. All these are from personal experience and have been used many times by a lot of grateful people of all age groups.

You do it all in the mind's eye.

What you are doing is getting rid of the effects and,, with each attempt, whatever it is *gets less and less* as you are working on it. This means that eventually with practice you can clear quite painful and traumatic things. Again, I am talking from experience.

Different people find different things suit them or suit different issues or even moods; so I have set out a variety of methods for you to try out. Again the choice is *yours.*

Be patient with yourself. Also be honest. You can afford to be because no-one need know anything because it ensures total privacy. Self-delusion and/or self-justification are negative. They will undermine your efforts and prevent you releasing important issues that need to be out of your system.

If you prefer you can do any of this with someone close to you for company, as long as they remain quiet for you. They might even have a try too while you are busy inside your own head and you can compare notes afterwards!

Think of this as a voyage of discovery. It will show you what you actually inflict upon yourself, and when it's 'gone' you know you are free of it.

Method 1.

This is the simplest, and is very enlightening as well as effective!!

- Sit somewhere quiet and comfortable.
- Start with a simple negative thought. Anything that starts with '*I hate….*' even if it's '*I hate going to work!*' It might even be '*I hate myself for…….*'
- Close your eyes and imagine something to write on and something to write with.
- Write up the complete *'I hate….*'sentence in your mind's eye.
- Get rid of it…rub it out, cut it, burn it, anything. But the whole sentence *must go.*
- Now write it **again** and get rid of it again…..
- And **again** until it just *will not* write!

How many times it takes to rub out or blow up tells you how much you really do hate what ever it is!! You can even write '*(S)he/they hate(s) me'* if that is a concern for you.

You really must make sure there is either no trace left, or it is impossible to write, otherwise it will stay with you. Remember those magnets!!

It is really useful in getting rid of deeply felt problems that you want to get rid of fairly quickly. **Especially if it's against yourself!** If there is something in particular bothering you, then write down on a piece of paper all the *feelings* you have about it. Useful starters are sentences that begin with '*I hate/despise/can't stand…..*' etc. Also '*I want….*' '*I need…*' - anything that reflects what is bothering you. And work through the list until they are all gone. If there are a *lot* of sentences, then try **Method 5**.

Once you've had some practice, you will find **Method 1** good for quickly getting rid of everyday negativity before it gets a hold on you! It's really useful for keeping you in good spirits despite petty irritations. If you are fed-up at feeling cold, unwell, anything, even get rid of the '*I'm fed-up being…*'! You'll feel the benefit, believe me!

Method 2 requires a little more time but, once again, it is very enlightening and most effective. It is good for anything troubling, frustrating, or distressing; long term issues like sense of loss or grief and often the remorse that goes with it, any recurring situations, - anything really. It's helpful if you are finding that a sentence in Method 1 is being obstinate! This will get rid of the issue related to it.

Try this method first on something that is a relatively minor sore point or concern to get the hang of it. It might be something that pops up just as you are reading this, or you are about to give it a try. Trust that first thought! Incidentally, if something is 'preying on your mind' ….it's always a good indication that it wants out!

Method 2.
Allow about half an hour or so.

• Make yourself comfortable in a quiet place. Sitting up is helpful so that you are less likely to fall asleep. Remember negativity makes you tired.
• Be patient and thorough with this; the benefits are definitely worth it.

You will already have the issue in mind even if it's in the back of it, so that will start the ball rolling.
• Now, as if you are picking up threads, quickly pick up as many feelings, thoughts and remembrances of the issue. *Don't explore them.* Just collect them.
• When you feel you have collected up the one's that come readily to mind, turn your mind to seeing if you can find or see your own feet *by **looking** carefully inside your head.* Give yourself time. If not, any other part of your body that you can see or feel. That will be a starting point - (or it might even be where the problem has lodged itself.)

In your mind's eye only:-
Assuming you can visualize or feel your feet:-
(any bit of you that comes up can be a starting point.)
• Wriggle your toes, rise up on them, lift one foot up and then the other. Feel all over them and under them.
• If any of this is difficult or there is something there that shouldn't be - *get rid of it*

You can use *anything*....you can't hurt yourself in your mind's eye. Try dissolving with light or even extra strength acid, cut and paste in a new bit, use an apple corer, laser, scalpel even, or massage heaviness or stiffness away etc. You can have someone (or several helpers) to help you if you like. Use your imagination and be thorough.

• What are you standing on?
• Get rid of it if it isn't nice or comfortable.
• Make your feet comfortable.
• Now work your way up your legs, back and front. Anything that shouldn't be there, get rid of it.
• Work slowly and carefully all over the front of the body, arms, elbows, hands, neck, throat, face, head/scalp shoulders, spine, back, waist and then down again to the feet.

• Remove anything you find anywhere that is not right or comfortable. It could be a 'something', a pain, an ache, heaviness, stiffness, tightness, a shadow, lumpy flesh that you would rather wasn't there, even a pimple or mole, anything, - it must go.

• If there is a pain or tenderness anywhere, imagine you have x-ray eyes. Now look inside where the pain is. If there is anything there that doesn't belong - even if it's a mist or shadow or funny colour - get rid of it. (You'll be surprised what you find!!). Be thorough, it needs to *go*! Remember, you can use anything or anyone's help.
• If it leaves a hollow or dent, get some healing paste to fill it up and get it back to normal. Make sure it really is as good as new!
If anything is being *really* difficult to get rid of, you can always quickly collect up the thoughts and feelings again and work on it again and repeat the process till it does go.
When your whole body is dealt with and quite clear, *stay in your mind's eye.*
• Now, in your *imagination* bend over & touch your toes, do a handstand /cartwheel/leapfrog and even a back flip. If you have 'cleared' properly, you'll manage all of them!! If there is any stiffness or fear, then clear it as before. You might have to have another go another time. But this *won't* happen if you've been thorough.

• Then, imagine having a nice run along a beach or grassy paddock in the sunshine feeling fit and full of life and then, *still in your mind's eye,* have a lovely hot shower and visualise all the worries, pain and discomforts from the problem are washing down the drain. When you are dried off and dressed comfortably, lie down to rest.
When you are ready to, open your eyes and you will feel brighter at the very least and usually as if a burden has dropped from you and your mind feels clear.

*****

Everybody is different. Therefore the results will be different.

They could be subtle and only show through changing responses in either a person or situation or an inner peace of mind. Some people actually feel the effects some time after. Suddenly a load seems to lift from them. This is usually with people who find it difficult to lay their burdens down because they feel they *should* carry them.

We are very good at hanging on to our emotional pain. We can even feel guilty for not doing any suffering when there is so much suffering in the world. But why add to it when you can suffer less and spread a little sunshine too?

By this time you should have a few issues in mind. It is to be hoped that you have made a note of some in *My Personal Notes* as you've read through the book. It's worth reading them through one straight after the other. There might be pattern there or a sequence that reveals areas in close relationships that have gradually built up un-noticed. In this way we can realize what issues or problems we are loaded up with. These subtly influence our relationships.

Viewing them collectively helps also to evaluate either a conflict situation or a whole relationship. These can be fixed if you want them to be. Both **Method 2** or the next, **Method 3** will bring about a positive and painless change for the better.

Method 3.

This is a goody if you have an issue or problem with a person. Past or present.

Try it first with a minor issue and work your way gradually towards difficult or complex ones over time. These can be dealt with in stages to make them more bearable if they are painful....but, remember you are not going to enter the pain, you are going to be *projecting* not 'feeling' and reducing it immediately.

• Once again, make yourself comfortable and close your eyes.
• In your mind's eye if possible conjure the person up in front of you - if too painful or you'd rather not, imagine a photo even if it's a really small one or their name! And be brave; they are *not* there really!
• Is there anything visible between you and the other person?
It could be something attaching you to them, or furniture, carpet etc, a shadow even.
• Get rid of it. Any method will do - (see above)
• If you have been burning to say something to them then do so. But let it all out! In any language you feel you want to use!!

You have several options at this point.

If you feel you can't go on facing them, you can dissolve them in some bright light and open your eyes. You will feel better. You might feel able to do it again at another time to see how things are and gradually work on them until the whole thing is resolved, which really would be good - for *you*.

This part can be either a continuation or you can come back to it later; or if you like, a regular way to deal with someone who is really being a pain on a regular basis because *they* are rooted in their issues and behaviour. It happens in the best of families or jobs. But they will improve once *you* are able sub-consciously to react less.

• The person is still in front of you. Imagine that what you feel is coming out of you towards them. It can take any form; so let it happen. Mist, a thread, anything. It might attach itself to them.

• Dissolve it from inside you, all along it and dissolve it where it's attached to them.

• Repeat this and then do the same with any other feelings you have on the issue until nothing comes from you.

• Now imagine that what *you* think *they* are thinking or feeling about the issue, is coming from *them.*

• Now dissolve it in the same way. Repeat this and with any other thought or feelings *you* think *they* have until nothing comes from them.

Two options again.

You can **either** then tell them the conflict is gone and dissolve them with bright light,

Or, - do this if you wish, or they are important to you, or close to you.

• Imagine you can fill yourself up with bright warm light.

• Imagine some coming up onto the palms of your hands.

• Hand this to the person in front of you and ask them to fill themselves up with the warm light too.

• Then hold their hands and feel the warm light flowing between you.

• Tell them that there is only love (or friendship or liking) flowing between you and that the conflict has gone.

• Thank them for helping you to clear the issues and then set them free in their own light. If it's a loved one give them a loving hug before you let them go.

• Stay in the image of the light flowing through you for a little while.

• If you are a spiritual person, imagine your guardian angel is enfolding you in his/her wings, making you feel loved and comforted. And the same for the other person.

When you are ready, open your eyes and relax.
You will feel good and often immense relief.

The people I have worked with who have done this warm light visualisation to finish off a session, even with the other methods, have all enjoyed it and felt even better.

Method 4.

This is a good chakra-clearing method that doesn't take very long.

It shifts surface negativity if you can't quite make up your mind why you are feeling down and/or some deep stuff if you can be particular about an issue.
It can also help shift physical pain by putting a 'pool' in the appropriate area too.

• Sitting comfortably with eyes closed.

You do the same thing with each chakra, starting at the **crown** chakra and working your way through each one till you get to the **root**.
Each time:-

- Place your hand lightly over the chakra area.
- Imagine there is a pool of water under your hand; imagine all the 'feeling fed-up'/worry/tension/tiredness/stressed-out/'under-the-weather' feelings are in the pool making it thick and dark. [If you have an issue or problem, pick up the threads of them as in **Method 1.** Put the bundle of thoughts (or a particular pain) in the pool of the appropriate chakra (eg: anger in the **root**) and imagine the water becoming darker and thicker.]
- Now take your hand away and imagine that, as you do so, the dark water gushes out from the front and back of the chakra until it's all gone. If it leaves a hollow or dent, put in some healing paste and make it as good as new and move on to the next one. If there is any residue left in the hollow, imagine rinsing it out with fresh spring water till it's all clear and then use the paste and heal it up.

If you find a lot of dark sludgy water in any of the chakras, repeat the visualizations until nothing comes out at all. It's surprising how much you could find and getting rid of it every last drop will make a big difference.

When all the chakras are clear, you can take a nice refreshing shower in your mind's eye as before and have a little rest before opening your eyes.

Or you can go through each chakra from **root** up to **crown** and fill them up with warm light before opening your eyes.
Or even better, both!

Method 5.

If you have a long or longish list of sentences, this is good and quite fun.

You can use a hold-all, a suitcase, or whatever takes your fancy.
We'll use the hold-all.

- Sitting comfortably with eyes closed.
- Imagine an open hold-all in front of you.
- One by one, pick up the sentences and put them into the bag. (or even people involved! Even an event. You can roll them up like a picture.)
- Close it and step back from it. Are you attached to it by anything or in any way? If so, whatever it is, cut it, dissolve it burn it, anything, but get rid of it.
- Now see if you can pick up the hold-all.
- It might too heavy, or be difficult to lift so ask for friends/firemen/soldiers - anyone to help raise it.
- Then get rid of the hold-all. Blow it up, dissolve it, put into an acid bath or a furnace or volcano - anything, but obliterate it!! - Whatever you like.
- Now do it all again. The holdall will gradually get smaller or more faded, or both.

• Repeat this whole thing until you just can't bring up the image of the bag!.
• Now brush your hands off mentally, relax and open your eyes.

Method 6.
This is pain or injury specific.

Pain is a signal for change. (*See* Chap. 17) The change here is to work positively on it. You can ask anyone you like in your imagination to help with any of it.
For any physical pain, ache or soreness, tenderness, bruising, stiffness etc:-
• Settle yourself comfortably and close your eyes.
• First imagine the pain has turned to liquid and imagine it running out till it's all gone.
• Then imagine you can look inside the part that is giving you the pain.
• Whatever you find there that shouldn't be there, get rid of it, dissolve it etc. If it is blank, rub out the blank or shine a light on it - something else will show itself. Ask for imaginary help from anyone you like if you need it.
• You can remove any organ, joint, bone etc and replace it with a new one.
• You can smooth a healing cream/oil/paste over any sore bits like joints or wounds.
• Keep clearing and healing the area in your mind's eye until it all looks healthy and normal inside. *You can come out and go back in to check there's nothing else as many times as necessary* till it remains looking normal.
• Fill the area with healing paste and make it all as good as new with no scars or rough skin on the outside. Mentally press the area to check all is healed.
• Repeat this by looking into the area from the back just as above.
• Finish off with either the shower, the run in the sunshine or the warm light visualisation (or something else calming and pleasant of your own choice for that matter) before resting and opening your eyes.
The pain will be easier. Sometimes it will even be quite minimal or even gone!

For those with chronic pain and/or several painful areas, (eg: in arthritis) it can be eased by working all the way through each painful joint/sore place with the above method. Visualising fresh new tissue, joints etc is good too. It will be worth the effort if you are having a bad day and fixed in a chair or bed anyway.

Doing this on a regular daily basis for on-going pain
helps keeps it under control.

Surrounding muscles that are tensed up will increase the pain. They frequently spasm to protect an injury or tense up because the body is positioned or held awkwardly to compensate the condition. Sitting in the same chair for long periods or just fear of moving in case or because it will hurt makes muscles stiff with tension and immobility too. Emotional tension *always* accompanies pain. Releasing it relaxes all body tissue.

This is very effective. For any injured or painful area, visualise putting the muscles and joints through their full range of movements *in your mind's eye.* As soon as you can't do a movement or anything hurts in the *mind*-body, clear it and try again until all the movements are easy to do. Being thorough in this way will relieve a lot of pain and tension and so is worth the effort. It can certainly help with breathing problems as well.

If you are really determined, it will be useful to take a mental note of the area and the energy centre related to it and the side of the body too. This could help you discover some emotional wound sitting in there holding the pain in place or deepening it. (This worked brilliantly with a lady who had severe persistent sciatica!) You can explore this possibility by looking back at the appropriate area in Section 1.

For particularly significant, strong, or deep problems, events or issues you can always follow one method with another. For example Method 5 can be followed by Method 2. This is always a good one to check whether there is any thing left. All you need do is re-think briefly the feelings and details and start the second method. Sometimes there is something tucked away if it's a persistent concern or issue.

******

Often with the release of negative emotional links, you feel tears coming on - let them flow - for as long as needed!! Because they are 'releasing' in themselves they will help immensely with the effectiveness of the link clearing. There is a substance in tears that has a slight sedative effect ie: it is soothing. You will feel heaps better afterwards; especially you men who scorn or are unused to tears. This is one time when letting go cannot come into the category of being 'feeble' or 'pathetic'! (This is negative thinking anyway!) There is necessity and pleasure in 'a good cry'!

******

For the Practitioner.

1) Method 1 can be suggested to your client, either for them to do later to clear blocked energy discovered during treatment, or suggest they try it out while treating them. This will help to clear the blockages as you go along. This works wonders on their energy system and facilitates the treatment you are giving, as you will discover.

2) Using these methods on yourself means you can speak from experience. Even more, it helps you enormously personally and as a healer. .

The fewer negative links you as a therapist or healer hold within, the less will connect *to* you *from* your client(s).

******

If having read through this section and you think it sounds far-fetched, nonsense or even rubbish, please do yourself a favour and give one method a try before you dismiss it. You will be surprised by what you visualise, if nothing else.

Having worked my way through my own experiences and issues, I still do this cutting of the ties for myself as forgotten issues, problems and new trying situations arise. It makes such a difference to my state of mind and general well-being, and my energy and positive outlook. This is why I have shared it with you as I do wish you to benefit too.

Once tried you'll know this works. You'll learn how to improve the technique the more you do it. The effort will be worth it. It's all down to you how much you put in.

******

Helpful tips.

1) A quickie that is helpful for any painful area: just imagine the pain has turned to liquid and visualise it running out till it's all gone. Repeat this till nothing pours out. This also works with worry, pouring out of your solar plexus, or tiredness, pouring out of your feet, or even distress, pouring out of your heart, or low self-esteem pouring out of your sacral centre. End with visualizing a beam of bright energy coming from your crown and flowing strongly down your body pushing any residual pain, tiredness or worry out of your feet. Very refreshing!

The anticipation, ie: the *idea*, of tiredness, pain, even taking a fall, will tense the muscles and deplete the energy system. Because the body rapidly responds to our emotions, the body's co-ordination is altered. Thus the body is primed before the event and receptive to further tension. We can readily see tiredness, pain and anxiety in people's 'body language', which reveals the weight of negative energy. Awareness of this helps us assess our physical circumstances better.

For the elderly or when recovering from illness, it's worth those 10-15 minutes with this visualisation to boost the energy after any chores or events that are tiring. Recovery time like this will keep you going but also, by being re-vitalised you will feel much better about yourself and your capabilities. Managing your energy like this will give you much more.

2)This is for the end of a stressful day so that your evening is more relaxed.

If you have a shower when getting in from work/shopping/visiting etc:-
Imagine all your irritations, worries and anxieties are seeping out of you and being soaped off with the suds and flowing down the drain leaving you free of them;
Or if you haven't time/opportunity find a few moments to *imagine* you are having a shower or are under a waterfall and all the stresses are flowing off you as above.

Here's how you can get your own body to help you, mind and body working physically together.

This next one is a helpful visualisation if you are particularly stressed with a churning tum and/or feeling panicky and upset. This anxious state means your *sympathetic system* is switched on by adrenalin.

3) Remember how the *parasympathetic system* counter-acts the sympathetic system? Well, stimulate the Vagus nerve supplying your whole digestive system by making a really conscious *mental picture* of your favourite food, or chocolate, assorted cream cakes or anything you *really* like. Conjure it up in your mind in great detail and imagine the look, the smell and then imagine eating it. This will calm that churning feeling as the vagus nerve then takes over and switches off the adrenalin for you! It'll give you the valuable time then to think more rationally about what is troubling you, or keep it at bay till you can deal with it.

******

To be able to help yourself by sending out less negative energy, therefore receiving less from others because you *attract* less of it, will definitely improve the quality of your life.

If we *feel* we are a failure, people treat us as if we are because that's what we *send out*. We all know a bad attitude attracts a bad attitude and that conflict of some sort is the result from the bad *feeling* coming from people. When someone is 'spoiling for a fight' verbal or physical, it's because they are full of negativity about something. The consequences are always hurtful or damaging in some way. It can be just as bad if it is simmering below the surface. It's better not to have anything they can subconsciously latch on to.

However, if you *are* attracting negative energy in a given situation or from someone, especially if it keeps happening, then *you* are bringing it to your *own* attention to be dealt with. *You* are actually trying to tell yourself so that you can *help yourself.* What better way than by letting the issue(s) go and releasing yourself from the negative hooks? Negativity is a tool after all.

You have the power to save yourself from emotional fragility. The choice is with you, for you now have the knowledge and the methods to help yourself.

Each new situation we encounter will bring a fresh measure of emotions; so how much better can we deal with things if we are not dragging the old ones along like a ball and chain to hamper us or even hold us back.

If you think of your body as a vehicle, a car you have been given, your energy as the fuel and your inner self as the driver, then how you drive it and maintain it is down to you. When getting into their own car, no-one automatically gathers up a bunch of negative bossy people to go with them, all trying to take over the controls or telling them how and where to drive!

But metaphorically you do if you stay emotionally attached to all the negative issues and memories of the past: they'll be your back-seat drivers and bossy passengers.

When we get behind the wheel, don't we like to decide how and where? Our handling of the controls, awareness of the road, its users and the state of our car determines what the journey is like. So metaphorically speaking life is about who is driving and how.

For that matter, do we metaphorically have a hand on someone else's controls?

> The greatest bonus from releasing the negative chains that hold our issues and problems in place is that *we release our own capacity to love.*

Until we do this releasing we do not realise what that capacity is or how little of it we really use. And the more we release, the greater are the benefits we gain from a different state of being. This really does come from a new way of experiencing the relationships around us. Relationships are about love and affection in some form; so realizing the full potential of them will make life really good. Also there would be more support and comfort in times of trouble and pain from those around you and vice versa. This will be a natural consequence, not something you have to ask for. How much better that is for everyone.

The choice is now up to you.

******

My Personal Notes

My Personal Notes

Chapter 22. There are no Rewards or Punishments, only Consequences.

We take for granted so many instances in which we have negative views and attitudes that we hardly notice them. Often we are so used to them we are unaware that they are in fact negative. If we can change our viewpoint to a positive one, our outlook will help us get things into perspective, see things in a better light. Clearer thinking will result!

One of the most common is that people think of much of life in terms of rewards and punishments….with punishment having the priority. This is because our fixation and conditioning over guilt and deserving to suffer predominates. This leads naturally to people requiring reward as a reason to **a**) compensate for the 'downs', especially of feeling guilt-ridden and **b**) as a way of coping with it. But all of this is negative and leads to negative thinking *against ourselves*.

> We need to have the positive view that there are really only consequences to learn from, and actually to enrich our lives.

We all have free will and choice. These are simply what *you* decide to do with, given knowledge and the conscious awareness that *you* bring to your life. But in using our free will and choosing a particular consequence, we need then to accept and deal with that result. *For consequences bring us experiences.* Experiences lead to knowledge and understanding of our lives and relationships after all. But to think of consequences with negative anticipation, and experiences negatively, is to reject the doors they open to us.

Free will and choice will determine *why* you have the experiences that come your way and how you live them or deal with them. However, it is our choice '*to take* or *not to take'* **responsibility** for any consequences of what we choose to do. That choice determines the way life unfolds!

Every action has a consequence. And there are not many consequences we are truly unaware of! We all know right from wrong. But if it is an unknown, we need to accept whatever the result is if we choose to go ahead!

In primæval times when things were much simpler, action was determined by need and risks were taken for appeasing hunger and survival. And like the animals, Man needed to be fully aware and alert to *survive* and he learned from that.

Life is much more complex for modern man. It can and does become overwhelming in its pressures and demands. However if Man blunders along without using his thinking abilities to consider the consequences but merely acts because he wants to, then, *added* to the natural consequences of that action will be a negative comeback from somewhere that he will not be prepared for.

> This can so easily lead to a negative cycle of 'conflict' and 'response' with things often out of control.

To think in terms of rewards and punishments is to immediately invite negativity. But by considering things in the light of consequences, we can 'review' things and do our thinking-best to prevent negative results. This will be to help ourselves from a positive view-point. Even if we have blundered and we often do of course, then even reviewing things after the event can help us cope with the result and, one hopes, accept and learn from it. Far better than looking to blame either ourselves or others in a negative frame of mind - and facing all the consequences of further negative energy and response!

Sophisticated man has added 'want' to need because Man discovered

the conscious power of will for Self.

This has become a thinking and/or unthinking selfish drive to impose the Will or self on others for one's own gain at the expense of and often detriment of others.

But freely choosing as a thinking human being to *be aware* and *accept* and *take responsibility* for the consequences of his actions, be they directed by desire or need is what raises Man above the animal kingdom. Knowing and facing what we are doing and especially *why*, makes us independent-minded people who can aspire to make life better by using the conscious power of will for Self properly. (It is a tool like any other). Therein lie hopes and dreams.

As long as we have assessed the situation and are prepared for the result, then self-blame and unworthiness will not come into the equation to add a further burden to whatever we may have to accept. We are freer to take responsibility and get on with life. Beating one's self up (or others) over it, helps no-one and is destructive. And then we don't get into the bind of self-pity and seeking solace and artificial comforts which end up giving us more 'consequences' we don't like!

We need to be in control of the consequences and not controlled *by* them.

Your strengths and weaknesses and character traits are the tools you have for the quality of your life. By *using* them you are not being mastered by them. They help you gain the experiences you need for knowledge and development. However it is your choice to use them, over-look them, reject them or neglect them....but the *consequences* are what you will live with. And negative ones will control *you*.

If you choose the negative aspects and ways of being, this invariably leads to inflicting this on others as well as yourself and a negative cycle is set up that inhibits and weighs down your mental and physical energy. But it *is* your choice! The consequences will be the *result* of that choice and *yours* to live with and cope with. *You* chose them. But negativity often makes us lose sight of what we can learn from the results. Blame gets in the way.

So the choice is also in your responses and invitation
to negativity from within yourself or from others.

It is the small consequences that make up the threads of life. They either combine to make a strong positive fabric to support us and give purpose to our lives or, the fabric is so fragile and weak from conflict and negativity that we feel vulnerable and afraid; 'victims' of life and circumstances, fate, a bad deal etc etc. By looking at the consequences of doing or not doing the small things of our lives we can see whether the day to day pattern is going to be strong or not.

Knowing about something is infinitely reassuring! So we need to ask ourselves *why* we are doing things that involve:-

- *negative consequences,*
- *self-blame* or *self-punishment.*

Since there are always two sides to everything, the options need to be considered. Self-punishment has two sides too. One is negative, because we have a low self-concept and the other, the positive is our inner self is trying to draw our attention to what we are involved in. That self-punishment can become such a habit that the positive aspect gets ignored and unable to come into the consciousness shows how oppressive negative energy can become.

Doing something we won't/don't like the result of.
Letting something happen that we don't like.

WHAT

- am I accepting/doing this for?
- am I preventing myself from doing because I'm accepting this?

WHY

- am I accepting/doing this?
- am I preventing myself/being prevented from doing it?

HOW

- am I accepting/doing this?
- am I preventing myself/being prevented from doing it?

- And 'Am I prepared to take the consequences?'

***

Because it is about consequences, we'll take a brief look at what many people in the West believe in, re-incarnation and the idea of karma.

To think of karma as a 'debt' or 'a punishment for past misdeeds' is to view it negatively - and that is unhelpful! Such a view puts us back to blame again and leads to either negative speculations, or, because it is unpleasant, just puts a full stop to the idea.

But karma is the sum of our responsibilities, our experiences and *how* we have lived them. Whether we have acknowledged any of it or not, it is the consequences of a life. In re-incarnation this becomes a reference book, a map of previous journeys and the negative energy we may have accumulated on the way.

Either way it is therefore, an individual's '*development plan*'.

The concept in re-incarnation is that the individual needs to take responsibility for those past experiences and resolve them by *learning from* and *understanding* the issues involved, then *leaving them behind* so that they are not repeated. This is positive thinking that will mean moving forward, which is the whole idea.

Because re-incarnation is about learning, the soul needs to learn everything possible about a given situation or issue or problem. This is why these seem to repeat themselves. But with each seeming repetition, the *equation* is different because the people involved are *different.* That's because we need to resolve all of it. This does not mean we should blindly repeat the same habits and negativities as before; it means we should look at what and why we are doing things so that we end up *knowing* what we are about in a positive way. To know is to be aware in the experience.

We do not bring the knowledge of past experiences with us; so we have to work it all out from the experiences and issues that arise in the present lifetime. They are the clues, the signposts to our development. They are not punishments.

But even if we do not believe in re-incarnation and karma, the same principles apply. Because our life's experiences are our development plan, we can choose to learn and move on, or lumber ourselves with all sorts of negative baggage and become dependent on it as a way of giving ourselves and others a hard time. This is how we learn ***how*** **to live**.

We develop as individuals (or souls, depending on your belief) through '**change**'.

The changes in life invariably come through adversity, or suffering of some kind or another. But we need that 'wake-up call' because while things are comfortable and reasonably uncomplicated, we are quite happy to jog along in a little rut or comfort zone. We become complacent and even lose fresh direction because nothing changes; it just repeats itself. There is no development. Our aspirations and will become weakened. This can happen in even a bad or poor environment as people accept and hunker down to an unpleasant or even brutal life and get in a motiveless rut.

But our inner selves that want us to grow up and develop draw to us what we need to wake us up. We set ourselves up through the actions we do or don't do. And 'change' to our lives is the consequence.

Change needs to be embraced because it brings fresh opportunity.

It needs to be taken good notice of and made real use of if we are to develop at all.

However, we *can* make changes by looking at what we have become *dependent* on. (The consequence of allowing our awareness to become dulled by habit, complacency, comfort or dull acceptance!) In this way we can make life more meaningful and lessen the ills and emotional pain.

For dependency is about power and control.

Modern society, in which ever country you can name, is about making people dependent. Nevertheless we can control our *own* lives by sorting out our own dependencies. This we *can* do because **our brain is our own**. And those that concern our energy system and the consequences in our social inter-change are from psychological and emotional sources. By asking ourselves '*What* or *who* controls me?', '*How* dependent do I want to be?', '*Why* am I dependent?', we can look at the consequences. And remember, dependencies and controls are on both sides.

Some emotional habits and dependencies.

- 'Bat and ball' negative situations.
- Being demanding/demanded of.
- Being manipulated/bullied/taken for granted/advantage of.
- Being a victim/of others/of habits /of dependencies.
- Emotional blackmail.
- Sense of empowerment from manipulating/bullying/taking advantage of others/situations.
- Needing proof/assurances of love/caring/affection, or guilt/remorse.
- Illness/being unwell/belief in feebleness/limited energy/strength.
- Parent/child relationships, (adult and in parenthood).
- The illusion of power over others.

Because it is in our relationships that most of our emotional exchanges occur, releasing that inner baggage will smooth relationships and the path of life immeasurably.

It's all about choices and responsibility for ourselves and above all, honesty *with* ourselves. Being honest with your conscious self is your private gift to yourself.

These determine the consciousness we have in the present.

Then we can assess things and choose what to do with the quality of our lives and, consequently, our *health*. Assessment is possible through understanding our emotional baggage, which is what has been revealed through our exploration here of our anatomy and the energy systems throughout this book.

The clues and answers to your life all lie within you.
This is what 'self-knowledge' is all about.

There are three useful key questions to ask yourself.

WHAT

- do I accept?
- do I accommodate?
- is the value I place on myself?

Then:-

WHY

If you are to understand the value you place on yourself, you also need to ask yourself about what you think you need from others.
For example :-
I need him - or her - or them:-
• to like/love me,
• be good to me,
• make life easier/better for me,
• understand me,
• appreciate me,
• answer my needs,
• support me.

Then ask yourself the same questions honestly, prefixed with for example: 'Do *I* like me….' or 'Am *I* good to me….'or 'Can *I* make life easier….' etc. The answer to all should be '*Yes'* because 1) You *should* value yourself. 2) *You* are helping yourself.

If the answer to any (or all) is '*No'*, then you really need to be honest with yourself and ask yourself *why*.
• 'Whose values of myself am I living by?
• 'Why do I actually need, believe or think I need these from another or others?'
Then you need to decide,
• 'What am I going to do about it?'
• 'What shifts am I going to make in my thinking, my belief in my own capabilities, and my vibration from those needs?'
• 'What are the consequences if I don't?'

Jealousy and envy are based upon lack of belief in our own value. Either can eat away at our emotional stability. This is self-destructive. It can spoil or even ruin a relationship. It hurts first you and invariably the person you love, or spoils what could be a harmonious situation. The vibration of negative need it sends out gives an undercurrent that makes things worse. This will create a negative cycle attached to the fear of not being good enough. Releasing the attachment to that idea and belief is the answer. Then jealousy or envy will not master *you,* or your life.

The choices you make will determine your dependency and/or empowerment. Self-value is to *be* yourself because you have learned and developed your own value system.

True Self-value is empowerment.

Being true to yourself is to choose to 'Self-value'. We lose our independence by depending on others for our identity.

We are creatures of habit. Accepting negativity and being negative is one of our strongest habits. We neither realise nor question this. We really need to become aware of it. By asking *why*, we can assess the levels we accept and live with. This will help us to control the quality of our lives. Acknowledging the sources of our issues and ill-health is half-way to doing something about both.

All experiences, especially *adversity,* show us *what we are made of.* We need this. Without them we do not know courage, adventure, triumph, strength of spirit, purpose or the ability to rise above life's terrors, traumas and pains. We do not know compassion or caring for the less fortunate and service to others. Above all, we would not know altruism, that greatest of all attributes that man can have. Therefore, nothing is a punishment, only a road to learning about ourselves and life.

Helping yourself through understanding and dealing with negative emotional energy means that the past can be the past. Carrying the past or re-living it in the present is to burden, even cripple oneself. Either way it is a dead weight. It means that you are going *no further* than the past or one day or one event in the past. This is an ending of the fullness that life has to offer. Perhaps we need to ask who wins, you or it? The future is facing us every day with all its newness. The consequence of staying trapped in the past is that your future will be filled with it too.

Ask yourself; *why* you are keeping the past with you? What is it achieving? What are you gaining? Do you get a sense of security by holding on to it? Is it perhaps at the expense of another? Are you punishing someone or yourself with it? Be honest with your answer to your conscious self. Your inner self already knows it.

Whatever the past holds, anything unpleasant or bitter; pain, sorrow, anger, or hatred, it is detrimental to yourself to go no further than those experiences. Help yourself by releasing yourself from them. Put the past where it belongs, behind you as a guide not a tormentor.

Then the present is freer and the future full of possibilities!

Your choices become your consequences.

All that happens to us or how we cope throughout life is from the *energy we emit.* And equally, whatever that energy is, positive or negative, *what we are doing with it.*

It is to be hoped that through this way of understanding our body and its functions and emotions we can learn to assess this for ourselves, just as much as discovering the quality of that energy. One of the hardest but most rewarding, not to say essential tasks is to come to understand **what** we are using it for and how we are using it....and why.

We misuse our energy if we are motivated by the Ego and the Will from our own neediness and issues.

We do this by giving it away, even throwing it (and our Will and Ego!) at others, being invasive with our energy, or giving it to people who either don't want it, or haven't asked for it. And importantly, we should assess what we are doing to *their* energy in the process too. We do ourselves no good by wasting this vital commodity, ours or theirs.

We need to use our energy constructively. Positive energy, and negative experiences used positively, can give us strength of purpose. Any motivation from the heart, the intuition and our conscious awareness will achieve this.

The best use, therefore, is for energizing ourselves for what we *need* to do, for *who* and *what* are really important to us. Then we really get the best out of life, and the people and situations we encounter will enrich our lives as they are meant to, from what we learn from them as much as the love, pleasure and enjoyment they have to bring. Then we too can bring these to their experiences in return.

These are important choices that only the individual can make. It is through them we can be truly the loving and caring people we need to be for each other - and ourselves.

We can easily assess what quality of life we really want by choosing whether or not to limit or even end the pulling power of our negative energy. If we don't choose to, then it is important to be honest with ourselves and ask; why do we want to attract negative responses and feed our own negativity from other people's?

We can convince ourselves that by holding on to our negative experiences and 'creations' we will make people treat us better, or that by giving these dark thoughts a 'shape' in our minds we can comfort ourselves and feel stronger. We are simply choosing a dark place to live in. This is to deny ourselves the warmth and inner expansiveness that comes from living free of them.

The body has 4 elimination systems for the stuff it doesn't want, or will make it unhealthy or has just plain finished with. The mind has one - YOU. So what are you going to do to help your mind and body to optimum health and vitality? And best of all, your heart, both its health, and its capacity to feel and know love?

Life is actually a journey towards the light through the darkness of negative energy that we all live with and accept. But growth always begins in the dark and the urge of all living things is to seek, grow towards and live in the light. 'Light' for us is in enlightenment, peace of mind, love and even happiness, all of which we seek.

This exploration of our physical and emotional beings has been to help that, journey, to work through and dispel the darkness we unconsciously carry inside us so that not only do we grow and develop, but come to actually live in the light as loving people.

Through this understanding of our *whole* selves comes
an *expansion of consciousness* that will enrich your life.

Now you have the knowledge and understanding, and ways of shifting negative energy to change those dark vibrations for the better, because you know ***why*** and ***how***. The *physical body* gives the *inner self* the most amazing ways of learning and experiencing a rich life, full of diversity and challenge. (Look closely at your own and you will see that this really is so.) Value it as the source of all knowledge and understanding.

Above all value it as the place of experiencing and learning to know what we all talk about, sing, write and shout about, want and desire most - *love*.

*****

Energy is generated by every living thing on the earth. Energy even lies at the very core of the earth, the magma that constantly bubbles up through volcanoes and heats geysers. Because we are on a living planet the combination of living energy is the essential connection for us all because it sustains all life. Every animal, plant and human being contributes and partakes of it in a constant communicating flow. Although we all have our own energy systems we are all part of the collective life force at all times. Just as air flows around us, so does the combined energy of the planet. We play our part in its quality through our emotions and emotional interplay. Grouped as we are in such close societies that is a considerable amount! In the huge cities around the world therefore, it is very intense.

We need to keep in mind that all living things respond and react to the energy around them. We *know* that all living things are open to loving energy and expand and grow in its influence, but close up and shrink away from the dark energy of anger fear and hatred.

Because it is invisible and intangible, we forget it is there and how powerful our generated energy is.

The question we need to keep asking is: 'What sort of energy are we living within and re-generating?'

We humans have the conscious ability to change our negative energy to positive and *be loving* people. It is a responsibility we all have. A responsibility to ourselves, those around us and ultimately to the wider world. We do contribute hugely to the collective life force of our planet.

We all really prefer love. How then can we not wish to live in the flow of as much positive loving energy as we can? Especially when it is ours to create.

Energy is the connection to everything. The essential connection for a good and healthy life is loving energy. We have an infinite capacity for it. We can all make use of that capacity. We can all determine the quality of our own life force. We have seen how each of us is the creator and generator of the energy we emit. Whatever the quality, it is the resource for our body and mind's vitality. Let us create and generate the best.

Full Glossary

Acidosis:... imbalance in ph of blood (acid/alkali)..acid levels up in Type I Diabetes, (pear-drops on breath) starvation, (anorexia) kidney failure, incomplete metabolism of fat , carbonic acid in blood, in respiratory illnesses or drug abuse. Symptoms are severe and life-threatening.

Antagonistic:...opposite action.

Anterior:…at or to the front.

Antibody:…destroys or de-activates bacterial invaders.

Antigen:…any foreign substance that activates immune system.

Arteriole:…small artery.

ATP:…**A**denosine **Tri**phosphate…(adenine, sugars & phosphates) main energy-carrying chemical made by body to collect and store energy for use in all cells.

Autonomous **N**ervous **S**ystem:…deals with all spontaneous and unconscious activity eg: internal organs etc.

Axon terminals:…axons end in little branches; each end in a minute bulb, a *synaptic knob*. These terminals (ends) store neurotransmitters.

Axon:…fibre that carries information *to* and *from* the nerve cell. (*white* matter) can be any length up to 3 feet.

Basal Metabolic Rate:…rate of metabolism ie: number of calories of heat per hour (calculated at rest) that keeps the body alive and well.

Bile:...mix of lecithin and bile salts produced in liver. Helps stimulate intestinal peristalsis to carry waste products away for elimination. Lack of bile lets fats coat other nutrients and prevents absorption. Protein is left undigested.

Bi-lobed:…(**bi-** = two)…having two lobes.

Blood Pressure:…pressure of blood through main arteries.

Bone matrix:…calcified rigid part of bone.

Broad Ligament:…a tough fibrous sheet that supports the uterus.

Bronchioles:…small airways branching off the bronchi in lungs.

Capillaries:…tiny vessels carrying fluids (blood or lymph) from tissues to arteries and veins.

Capsule:…sac containing fluid.

Catabolism:…release of energy into cells from breakdown of fats.

Catalyst:…chemical that creates a chemical change between others but remains *un*changed itself. Enzymes are catalysts.

Cerebellum:…hind brain controlling body movement & stability.

Cerebral:…to do with the Cerebrum.

Cerebrum:…higher conscious brain.

Cholesterol:…lipid steroid; most abundant in body. Used to synthesise steroid hormones (eg: testosterone) and bile salts.

Chyme:…partly digested stomach contents passed out to duodenum for pancreatic juices to work on.

Clavicle:…collar bone.

Colloid:…thick fluid.

Combustion:...burning of oxygen & sugars to create heat & energy.

Components:…contents making up an item.
Connective tissue:…fine tissue that binds and supports; holds specialised groups of cells together; most widespread tissue in body.
Corpus callosum:…central mass of white nerve fibres connecting the two hemispheres of the brain.
Corpus: *(Latin = body)*.... body or mass of specific cells.
Corpuscle:…literally, 'small body'.
CRH:…Corticotrophin **R**eleasing **H**ormone.
Cytoplasm:…soft gel round the nucleus of a cell containing all its necessary molecules.
Degenerate:…to break down.
Dendrites:…(*dendro* = tree) Many-branched filaments extending from nerve cell body linking neurones to one another.

There is a tiny *gap (synapse)* between the endings of neighbouring dendrites. Electrical charge from neural activity, jumps this gap to connect neurones to pass on the information they carry.

Diagnose:…from Gk...*Dia* = from… *gnosis* = knowledge.
Diffusion:…to pass directly through the cell walls. (always from an area of *greatest* concentration to one with less)
Dilation:…widen.
Disintegrating:…breaking up.
Dispersal:…spread out to other areas.
Duct:…tube carrying substances out of an organ.
Ductless:…has no collecting tube (duct) to carry substances to other areas.
Efferent:…outgoing (nerve); transmits impulses away from source.
Electrolyte:…ionises solution to enable it to take an electric current.
Ellipsoid:…slightly flattened oval shape.
Embryo:…developing infant from fertilised egg up to 3rd month.
Emulsifying:…fat dissolved in water.
Engorgement:…filling up.
Epithelium:…outer layer; contains no blood vessels.
Equilibrium:…even balance.
Excretion:…getting rid of waste products.
Fascia:…deep = around organs and muscles etc; superficial = just under skin. Fatty insulating protective tissue that carries blood & lymph vessels & nerves.
Fibrils:…very fine fibres.
Fimbriæ:…fringed edges of fallopian tubes.
Fluctuating:…changing back & forth.
Fœtus:…developing child from 3rd month till birth.
Fornix:…arch.
G proteins:…protein passing signals from eg: hormones to receptor cells.
Ganglion/a:…area of grey matter of un-myelinated fibres.
Glucose:…simplified sugar. Small enough molecules for absorption.
Grey matter:….nerve cells where messages are received, interpreted and responses transmitted.

Hæmoglobin:…protein with iron in red blood cells that carries oxygen.
Hormonal:…hormone activity.
Hormone:…alters the physiological activity of target cells.
Hyper-:…above … more than.
Hypo-:….under … less than.
Hypochondria:…intense chronic interest in one's health/belief that one is suffering from ill-health.
Hypoglycæmia:…Low Blood Sugar Levels:-
hyp**o**...Below/Under….. hyp**er..**Above.
Hypophysis:…below body of brain.
Hypothalamus:…control/relay centre for neural messages to and from the body and the …………………..endocrine system/cerebrum…(some seratonin also found here.)
Impulses:…nerve messages that travel along nerve fibres to initiate action.
Inhibit/inhibition:…prevent/ put an end or stop to.
Initiates:…starts off/sets in motion.
Inteferon:…protein that inhibits virus reproduction.
Inversion:…tucked up inside
Involuntary:…not under conscious control.
Leucocytes:…white blood cells that kill viruses & some tumour cells.
Leukocytes:…white cells..collective name for five types with various functions, including lymphocytes.
Libido:…sex drive.
Lipoid:… pertaining to fats & oils.
Lobules:…small lobes.
Lobules:…small lobes.
Lunar Phases:…changes of the moon.
Lymph:…specialised fluid between cells that absorbs excess fluid and proteins and returns them to blood stream via the lymphatic vessels.
Lymphocytes:…2 types. **T**; attack infected/cancerous cells & **B**; produce antibodies.
Masses:…groups of cells for a particular function.
Meiosis:...distribution of chromasomes (divide into 2 equal halves).
Meninges:…semi-transparent membranes or thin skins covering the brain.
Menses:…monthly bleeding in women; release of endometrium (lining of uterus) when fertilization has not taken place.
Metabolic:…chemical changes that manage energy throughout body.
Molecule:…2 or more atoms joined together.
Mucosa:…mucus membrane; lining of all cavities.
Myalin:…fatty insulation formed from special neuroglia cells to conduct impulses.
Myriad:…many.
Nerve Pathways:…Essential that these are strongly established. Sufficient time in infancy for the full stages in crawling and free toddling is needed for this to occur. This establishes the dominance of one hemisphere by age 5, so that the **ear, eye, hand** and **foot** are dominant on either the left *or* right. This ensures good *motor skills*. These early stages are therefore essential and are best not shortened, discouraged or inhibited.

Nerve:…bundle of axons.
Neucleated:…containing the neucleus.
Neural:…to do with nerves & their activity.
Neuroglia:…(*Neuro* = nerve..*glia* = glue)connective nervous tissue that surrounds & supports nerve endings (neurones) with various functions.
Neuron:…nerve cell **body**; does not sub-divide (*grey* matter).

3 parts:-

- Nucleus and proteins for growth/function; renewal of damaged axons and dendrites.
- **Axon hillock**. Tapered portion which develops a thread-like process, called,
- The **initial segment**; (*grey* matter) from which axon grows.

Neurone:…complete nerve cell body plus its axon and dendrites.

Neurone *sending* impulse = presynaptic neurone. (pre- = before)
Neurone *receiving* impulse = postsynaptic neurone. (post- = after)
Grouped knots of these neurones are called **Ganglia**. (*ganglion* = knot) (*see* basal ganglia)

Neurotransmitter: chemical substance released by neuron to communicate with the next one: changes the *electrical* impulse into a *chemical* one and allows it to jump the *synaptic cleft*, and so transfer the information to the neuron.

Damage to nerve cell body………irreparable. Neuron and axon die.
Damage to axon hillock/axon(s)…repair/re-growth.
Damage to dendrites……………..repair/re-growth.
Severing of axon(s)………………if *no link to cell body* nucleus, axon dies

Addictive substances can affect Synapses. (Staggering while drunk for example!)This prevents or blocks homeostasis especially long term abuse

Nocturnal eneursis:…bed-wetting.
Nodes of Ranvier:…gaps in myalin sheath for nerve impulse to jump to increase speed
Nucleus:…living part of cell where cell activity takes place.
Œsophageal:…to do with the œsophagus; the food pipe.
Oogonia:…primitive female sex cells.
Optic Nerve:…large nerve from eye to brain.
Osmosis:…fluid/molecules can pass through membrane one way but not back.
Ovum:…egg….**ova:**…plural.
Oxidizes:…addition of oxygen
Pathogens:…micro-organisms causing disease.
Peristaltic: ...muscular action to churn and move digestive contents along.
Permeability:…having the ability to let substances pass through.
Phagocytes:…white blood cells that surrounds & digests pathogens.
Phagocytosis:...(Phagocytic (Gk. = 'Cell-Eating') ingestion of bacteria by specialised white cells (phagocytes).
Plexus:…network of nerve centres with converging and diverging fibres.

Polycystic:...many cysts, swollen pockets filled with fluid where ova usually ripen.
Posterior:...At or to the back.
Postganglionic:…taking impulses away from a ganglion.
Psychosomatic:…symptoms caused or made worse by emotional belief in them.
Receptor:…specialised cell a substance binds to.
Receptors:…cells that receive specific chemicals. Numbers increased & reduced as needed.
Respiration:…exchange of oxygen & carbon dioxide as waste through lungs via blood.
Retention:…holding back.
Reticular activating system:..relay network of nerves in Brainstem for consciousness
Sacule:…little sac.
Sagittal:…side view.
Saline:…salt in solution (eg: water).
Schwann cells:…name for coils of myalin between nodes of Ranvier.
Secretion:…useful fluid product made and released from a gland or cell.
Secretory:…has the ability to secrete specialised substances.
Seminiferous:…to do with/pertaining to semen.
Seratonin:…neuro-transmitter that controls mood, induces calm. Counter-acts adrenalin response.
Sign:…evidence that can be seen, eg: swelling, rash etc.
Sinus:…collecting place for fluids.
Sinusoid:…small sinuses.
Skeletal:…to do with the skeleton/bones.
Spermatazoa:…mature sperm cells which swim towards ripe ova.
Spermatogonia:…stem cells that become sperm cells.
Spermatozoon:…sperm cell with no tail (tail released once inside ovum.)
Spermogenesis:…production of sperm cells.
Sphincter:...circular muscle at a natural opening that opens and closes when stimulated to let substances in & out.
Stimuli:…plural of stimulus.
Stimulus:…a trigger to start activity.
Symptom:…change in body's function that indicates illness, eg: vomiting, sweating etc.
Synaptically:…crossing of impulse over a gap to pass messages from neurone to neurone.
Synthesises:…forms substances by linking several molecules into specific groups.
T cells:…white cells matured in the Thymus gland.
Thalamus:…area of grey matter (nerve cells) under brain for senses/emotions/arousal. (some seratonin also found here.)
Trachea:…(tra..*kee*..a)…wind pipe from throat to lungs.
Type 2 Diabetes:…The overworked sugar metabolism systems triggers a reduction in the insulin hormone receptors in cell membranes, so Insulin production is thus decreased Glucose molecules are therefore not able to be diffused into the cell for its metabolism and the glucose therefore remains un-used in the blood. The cells become starved and full function is impaired.

UV:…Ultra-Violet.
Vacuoles:….little membrane sacs to hold or store substances.
Vagus nerve:…large many-branched nerve supplying the digestive system. *see* **ANS**
Vascular:…pertaining to or well-supplied with blood vessels.
Ventricle:…chamber.
Vibratory:…having the ability to vibrate and give off sound waves.
White matter:…fibres carrying messages in electrical impulses to and from brain and body.
Zygote:…fertilised ovum. ie: union of male and female gamete.

******

Index.

Bibliography

Anatomy & Physiology. Thibodeau Patton 3rd edition pub: Mosby
Aids to Anatomy & Physiology for Nurses. Katharine F. Armstrong, SRN SCM DN(Lond) 6th edition. pub: Ballière, Tindall &Cox
Applied Physiology . Samson Wright 7th edition. Oxford Medical Publication
Ballière's Nurse's Dictionary. Barbara Cope. 15th edition
Principles of Anatomy & Physiology. Tortora Grabowski 7th edition, pub: Harper Collins
Schafer's Essentials of Histology, ed: H. M. Charleton 14th edition pub: Longmans, Green & Co
The Human Body, Marshall Editions Ltd 1989